DON'T WORRY:

MY MOM IS THE TEAM DOCTOR

THE COMPLETE GUIDE TO YOUTH SPORTS INJURY AND PREVENTION FOR PARENTS, PLAYERS, AND COACHES

DON'T WORRY:

MY MOM IS THE TEAM DOCTOR

THE COMPLETE GUIDE TO YOUTH SPORTS INJURY AND PREVENTION FOR PARENTS, PLAYERS, AND COACHES

CAROL FREY, MD, AND JACOB FEDER

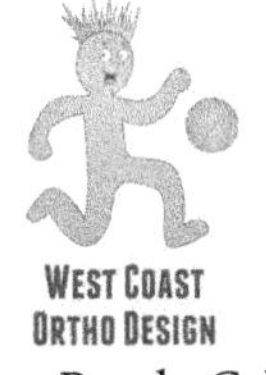

Manhattan Beach, California

Don't Worry: My Mom is the Team Doctor
The Complete Guide to Youth Sports Injury and Prevention for Parents, Players, and Coaches

On the cover, coauthor, Jacob Feder, age 9. Photo from the private collection of Carol Frey, MD.

Photography by Ralf's Photography, El Segundo, Calif.; and Carol Frey, MD. West Coast Sports Medicine Foundation, Manhattan Beach, Calif.

Because of the dynamic nature of the internet, any web addresses or links contained in this book may have changed since publication and may no longer be valid. The views expressed in this work are solely those of the author and do not necessarily reflect the views of the publisher or their agents.

Disclaimers: Trademarks of products, services, and organizations mentioned herein belong to their respective owners and are not affiliated with the publisher. The information, ideas, and suggestions in this book are not intended as a substitute for professional medical advice or official policy governing youth sports. Before following any suggestions contained in this book, you should consult your personal physician for specific information about your condition. Neither the authors nor the publisher or their agents shall be liable or responsible for any loss or damage allegedly arising as a consequence of your use or application of any information or suggestions in this book.

For information, address the publisher:
West Coast Ortho Design
Carol Frey, MD
1200 Rosecrans, Suite 208
Manhattan Beach, CA 90266
(310)416-9700
www.DontWorryMyMomIsTheTeamDoctor.com

Paperback ISBN: 978-0-9909011-1-2
Kindle ISBN: 978-0-9909011-0-5
Epub ISBN: 978-0-9909011-2-9

Library of Congress Control Number: 2014954629

Printed in the United States of America.

10 9 8 7 6 5 4 3

To James Richard "Dick" Frey, a graduate of Banning High School, where he lettered in track, baseball, and basketball. His shot put record stood at Banning High School from 1939 to 1976. He was described in the *Los Angeles Times* in 1940 as the "outstanding player of the strongest basketball league in the city set up—that's the honor earned by Dick Frey, high scoring center of Phineas Banning in Wilmington. To be the outstanding player, of the outstanding team, in the outstanding league is quite an accomplishment."

Dick Frey received the Helms Athletic Foundation Athlete of the Year Award in 1940. He played on the All-City and All-Southern California Board of Basketball first team in 1938, 1939, and 1940. He was the CIF basketball player of the year in 1940. He received a scholarship from USC to play baseball and/or basketball and chose basketball.

He was a decorated veteran of World War II, a scientist, an elite-level athlete, and my father. I dedicate this book to him and to all the scholar athletes who follow his path.

Contents

Forewords

By Holly McPeak and Christopher St. John "Sinjin" Smith

Holly McPeak: If you consider all that has happened in the last forty years since Title IX passed, there has been an explosion in girls' sports. There are more than ten times more girls playing high school and college volleyball than boys.* This has caused a huge increase in the number of kids—boys and girls (especially)—playing youth and club volleyball.

Just as in other sports, parents are spending a bunch of money on club sports, equipment, and personal trainers. This does not even include the time they spend driving their kids back and forth to early-morning and faraway tournaments.

There are higher expectations for kids in competitive sports today than existed in the past. Kids have to be mentally and physically tough to progress through the levels of their sport and have longevity. To make it in any sport, as in life, you have to give 100 percent.

I wasn't the tallest girl on my volleyball team, standing five feet seven, but I was always there to compete at the highest level and make an impact. I have never let anyone or anything stand in the way of obtaining my dreams. Success not only depends on sport-specific talent or size, but on coaches, trainers, teams, off-season training, working on the fundamentals of the sport, teammates, opportunity, your parents, toughness, love of the game, and a good medical team if you get injured.

Don't Worry: My Mom Is the Team Doctor not only walks you through the rigors and risks of youth sports but helps you deal with your injury while you are on the sidelines. Just like errors and mistakes in the game, almost all players suffer an injury at some point in time. An injury, just like a bad play, does not define you. This book will help you avoid unnecessary risk, train properly, recognize pain, and play without fear and for the joy of the game.

As participation in volleyball has increased over the past two decades, the number of volleyball-related sports injuries has increased. Luckily, the young athlete is basically healthy and able to withstand the physical stress of competitive sports with remarkably few injuries. Keeping in mind that kids often participate with a degree of enthusiasm and competitive spirit that often exceeds their physical abilities and skills, this is a feat.

Dr. Frey has written a book that is easy to understand and approaches all aspects of youth sports injuries. With discipline, hard work, and taking good care of yourself, anything is possible.

Holly McPeak's first appearance on the pro beach volleyball scene was in 1991. McPeak was named All PAC-10 and All-NCAA Team in 1990 and led her team to the NCAA Championship. She was voted NCAA Freshman of the Year in 1987. All totaled, she has had seventy-two career titles. She is a three-time Olympian, NCAA champ in 1990, 2004 bronze medalist, five-time MVP, and seven-time best defensive player in the AVP (Association of Volleyball Professionals). Perhaps no other woman player has had more of an impact on beach volleyball's rise to international prominence.

[*The National Federation of State High School Associations reported that close to 404,000 girls participated in high school volleyball compared to around 50,000 boys in the 2009–2010 school year.]

Sinjin Smith: Volleyball, including beach volleyball, is one of the fastest-growing sports in the world. We are seeing an increase in the size and number of club-level teams for young athletes, high school, and college programs. It is exciting to be part of the expansion of a sport that I love and to have had the longevity and success to help it grow.

I have played for one of the all-time great coaches in any sport, Al Scates at UCLA, who not only knew how to win but how to get the best out of his young players. Even if he did not have the best talent during the season, he was able to figure out a way to get the best out of each individual to get a win. He had a sense of and confidence in the kids he coached and was never afraid to pull an unseasoned player off the bench to play at a critical time.

The young players who had the privilege to play for this positive coach have almost all gone on to success in volleyball and anything else they wanted to do. He taught us how to give 100 percent all the time, respect your opponents, never give up, focus on the next play, inspire your teammates, practice like you play, and even if you have the lead, don't let up.

The lessons I have learned in volleyball have stayed with me through life and my career. These lessons came from the sport, being part of a team, from positive coaching, and hard work. With the growth of any sport, there is an increase in injuries. The increase in injuries may be because there are more kids playing, more exposures, more competition, and perhaps more pressure to do well. Most players will have a few injuries that keep them on the bench for a few games. It happens. In sports such as volleyball, there are a lot of ways to get hurt.

Almost every athlete I know has played with pain at some point in time. But to have longevity in a sport, you need to be serious about taking care of your body. We know so much more today about injuries and how to deal with them so they don't become worse, which means you will be able to compete much longer. It is important to recognize an injury, seek appropriate treatment, and make sure you come back slowly as you return to the sport.

Don't Worry: My Mom Is the Team Doctor is a practical and easy guide through the maze of youth sports injuries. The young athletes, their parents, and their coaches will find practical tips and suggestions that they can use to recover from or prevent an injury. Dr. Frey takes complex medical information and distills it into easy and interesting material that will keep you in the game.

Christopher St. John "Sinjin" Smith is regarded as one of the greatest players in beach volleyball history. He is an Olympian and World Champion and became the first player to reach one hundred career open victories, and still remains atop the leaderboard to this day with 147 recorded victories, not to mention countless numbers of other wins at tournaments throughout the world. He has been honored for record-breaking accomplishments in the sport of beach volleyball and for dedication and commitment to developing the game for future players. In 1996, Sinjin was a member of the first American team to qualify for the debut of beach volleyball as a full medal sport at the 1996 Atlanta Olympics.

He has served as president of the Association of Volleyball Professionals, as a board member of USA Volleyball, and as president of the FIVB's Beach Volleyball World Council. Smith currently is a member of the FIVB Beach Volleyball Commission, presiding over the sport in 220 member countries for the Olympic games and the FIVB World Tour. He is also a past member of the board of directors of the Big Brothers, Big Sisters organization and the United States Youth Volleyball League (USYVL). He is a member of the International Hall of Fame and the UCLA Hall of Fame as well as being inducted into the Catholic Youth Organization Hall of Fame in 1998.

Introduction

> From Jacob Feder: It all started on my club basketball team in fourth grade. Kids were getting injured left and right, whether it was the occasional break of a bone or the more common ankle sprain. I was included in the bunch, but while others were scrambling for the latest web page on how to treat their injuries, I was getting first-class treatment courtesy of my parents, who were, are, and will continue to be doctors.
>
> Seeing this divide between my road to recovery and that of my fellow basketball players, I felt compelled to let my parents know whenever there was an injury out on the court. I would tell my teammates, "Don't worry, my mom is a doctor." Of course, I was able to take care of some of their lesser ailments, but when things got serious, my mom was the person to call.
>
> So when my mom and I started putting this book together, coming up with a title was obvious. You don't have to worry. My mom is the team doctor, and she can advise you too. Okay, Mom, your turn.

My son Jake has always been curious about medical issues, and I was happy to jump in to assist when his teammates were in pain. My son knows more about youth sports injuries than many trainers, in fact. I am happy to have him with me in collaborating on this book.

My business is treating injured athletes, and I have been doing this for over two decades. In the last few years, I have noticed a marked increase in the number of very young athletes, some as young as five, with adult-type injuries.

It is common for the parents to want the injury explained to them in language that they understand—a practice they often do not get in an emergency room. They want to know what an injury to the growth plate is, how long their kid will be out of play, when their child can start practicing again, and does their little player "really" need a cast.

It is my job, and my mission, to explain things so that the parent and the child understand the injury, the treatment, and the terms for return to play. I am not aware of another source to refer parents, coaches, and players that describes all the parameters of youth sports injuries.

That's why I wrote this book. I want to explain athletic injuries so parents, young athletes, and their coaches can understand what happened, what happens next in treatment and recovery, and how rehabilitation will get the athlete back on the field—and when.

My son Jake has contributed to the book by bringing the experiences of injured young players to these pages. He has interviewed countless young athletes as they related their experiences and thoughts at the time of injury, navigated through the emergency room, visited the specialist, wore their cast or brace, rehabilitated their injury in physical therapy, sat on the bench with the coach ignoring them, and then returned to play.

Young athletes have a perspective on their injuries that is worth listening to. Their stories may help your child understand and rehabilitate—and prevent—injuries.

Remember, even Kobe sits on the bench with a knee injury, Shaq with a toe injury, and Joe Theisman with a broken leg. It's all part of the game, but it doesn't need to be career ending.

If you have school-age children, chances are you spend your weekends sitting in a fold-up canvas lawn chair in the shade, pacing the sidelines, trying to get comfortable in the bleachers, and certainly playing chauffeur to kids' practices and games.

Your kids are among more than thirty million kids playing organized sports in the United States. About three-fourths of families with school-age children have at least one kid who plays organized sports.

Whether it's on an elite football team, with a performance ice skating troupe, on a Pee Wee baseball team, or with a parent-coached soccer league, more and more kids are playing sports (and I emphasize the word *play* because sometimes we parents get too exuberant in expressing the importance of sports, and that's part of the problem I address shortly).

Millions more kids play sports than in all college divisions and professional athletes combined. Although participation by boys has increased 10 percent and more in the last few decades, participation by girls has increased 40 percent, according to the National Federation of State High School Associations.

We sports docs think kids are too inactive, which is leading to record levels of childhood obesity, but we also are making the case that kids are playing sports at record numbers and suffering injury in record numbers. Both trends are accurate. We can address the issues of inactivity and injury.

Yes, sports participation can improve a child's physical fitness, confidence, weight control, coordination, self-discipline, and teamwork—a message from Safe Kids USA and the Centers for Disease Control and Prevention (CDC). Even the national agenda supports activity. The decades-old President's Council on Physical Fitness and Sports still promotes "60 Minutes or More a Day, Where Kids Live, Learn, and Play."

First Lady Michelle Obama's "Let's Move" initiative is promoting healthy eating and active living at a time when schools have cut back on recess, and the nation is literally expanding in an explosion of overweight and obesity among children. Not to mention the skyrocketing rates of diabetes we doctors are seeing in obese children, when we never used to see type 2 diabetes in kids.

Youth sports can be a shining example of what works for kids in keeping them active and showing them lifelong habits around partnership, leadership, collaboration, and physical activity.

Yet kids are getting injured while playing sports. In fact, a third of all kids' injuries are sports related. High school athletics account for an estimated 2 million injuries, a half million doctor visits, and thirty thousand hospitalizations every year. Children ages five to fourteen account for nearly 40 percent of all sports-related injuries treated in hospitals (Powell and Foss 1999).

As a mom of student athletes, it is good to see the increase in the number of kids participating in sports. My sons are active participants in many sports, including karate, Little League, youth basketball, club and high school basketball, club and high school volleyball, and tennis.

These sports have their own sets of pros and cons. Basketball is fast-paced, technical, and indoors. On the flip side, aggressive parents are confined to an indoor gym, using colorful language, and fights in the stands erupt in proximity to the players. Baseball is truly the "boys of summer" sport, along with lawn chairs, nice weather, good food, teamwork, and big plays. The cons are that some may consider baseball slow-moving and prone to overuse of the throwers (and risk for injury), with aggressive parents who coach the game from the stands and threaten the umpire for sport.

Karate is a sport of discipline and patience. The negative is that karate is a sport of discipline and patience. Volleyball is a team sport with jumping and aerobic skills that can be enjoyed indoors and outdoors. It is exciting to see that volleyball is one of the fastest growing sports for girls. The negative may be that it is an expensive club sport, which some may consider elite. Tennis is a wonderful individual sport that can be played at all ages. The negative is that the parent is often the primary organizer and promoter of the sport for the child, and families may need to join a country club and hire a private coach.

Regarding football, I will save that discussion for an entire chapter.

Organized youth sports is wonderful for team building, discipline, exercise, weight control, friendships, fun, and something to do so you stay out of trouble! Studies have shown that kids who play sports stay in school longer and are less likely to do drugs or join gangs (Pate, Trost, Levin, and Dowda 2000). Wow, there is so much to say about the benefits of organized sports.

My older son, Jake, has played on several elite club teams and on his high school basketball and volleyball teams. My younger son is still in Little League and youth basketball. I have gotten up at 5:00 a.m. to drive a hundred miles for tournaments, stayed in cheesy motels, eaten team meals in diners, and had four-hour waits between volleyball matches. I have developed close friendships with the parents on the team, watched my sons make friends, and admired them as they develop discipline and skills.

I have seen my sons get injured and learn more about anatomy and physical therapy terms than any kid should. When your son tells you he needs an MRI and possibly a short leg walking cast for a growth plate injury in the fibula, perhaps he has had one too many injuries. No, wait, his mom is the team doctor!

However, with my doctor hat on now, I have to report that the number of sports injuries has increased at a higher rate than would be expected or is proportional to participation. I wonder if overly exuberant (read that *pushy*) parents underestimate the risks involved with kids' sports.

In my view, elite-level athletes seem to be getting younger and younger. NBA draft picks who don't finish college are old news. Now teenage players are being closely followed on Max Prep, ESPN Top 100, Gatorade Fab 50, and other sites. Not only are more of our children playing organized sports, but they are also participating at a younger age, specializing sooner, and playing with more intensity. If fourteen-year-olds are being scouted by D-1 colleges to play football and basketball, how can we blame the kid (or the kid's parents) for specializing at an early age?

As competition increases, the pressure on young athletes increases. The striving for athleticism, physical ability, and mental toughness is huge. For athletes who want to compete at an elite level, training in the off-season is required. Pressure to compete at a high level comes from athletic directors, trainers, coaches, parents, teammates, and the athletes themselves. There is an increase in the amount of training, intensity, and frequency of performance required to play sports at that level.

Furthermore, parents spend a bunch of money on equipment, personal trainers, and club sports. There are higher expectations for kids in competitive sports today than existed years also. Kids have to be mentally and physically tough to make it through the various levels of their sport. Success not only depends on individual talent but on parents, coaches, trainers, teams, teammates, and the sports medicine specialist (if the child is injured).

The young athlete is generally very healthy and able to withstand the rigors of competitive sports with remarkably few injuries. This is especially surprising considering that kids are often playing with a degree of enthusiasm and competitive energy that often exceeds their physical attributes and technical skills. How many of us, for example, have yelled our lungs out as our Little Leaguer smacks one out of the park and runs his little legs off rounding the bases getting to home plate and misses second base? Or runs toward the wrong goal in soccer? Or never seems to dribble the basketball without it hitting her shoe and bouncing out of bounds?

Many of these young athletes are participating in a sport that is new to them, or they are in full-throttle competition after only a short preseason. Coaches often find that they must skip some aspects of physical preparation in order to teach sports fundamentals and prepare a group of novice players to function as a team.

In addition, many young athletes participate in more than one sport with no period of recovery or rest between seasons. Some kids may participate in one sport, but combine school and club play with little or no rest between. This is a formula for injury. And that's why you are reading this book.

Let me pose some vital questions I address in this book (and give a short answer here):

- **Kids are different. Does an increased level of sports participation affect the immature body differently than the adult body?** Yes, the increased participation can affect the growing bones at an area called the growth plate, which adults do not have.
- **Do kids have the same injuries as an older athlete?** Yes, but they also have their own unique set of injuries, such as fractures of the growth plates, that adults do not have.
- **Does intense training or overtraining have any other long-term effects?** Yes, overtraining can lead to injury to the growth plates if symptoms are ignored.

- **Are certain sports more dangerous to kids than others?** The statistics tell us this is true, but you may be surprised which ones are the most dangerous.
- **Do kids specialize too soon?** Quite simply, yes.
- **Should children train differently than an adult?** No question about it, yes. But the basic principles of conditioning still apply.
- **How do children deal with "sports" injuries?** Kids are resilient. The biggest barrier to their coming back to play is regaining their confidence and mental toughness. This is a bigger problem with older kids.
- **What is the psychological effect of injury on the young athlete?** Just as heartbreaking as it is for older athletes. This is especially true if the kid identifies himself or herself as an athlete.
- **Can too much too soon lead to early burnout or other negative consequences?** Yes. I'll advise you on how to strike the right balance.
- **Would I let my son play football?** This is a very personal decision. We will weigh the risks versus the benefits.
- **Are parents getting too involved in play on the field?** Yes, and that's why I address this in the very first chapter. This is *not* your father's sandlot pickup game!

The Facts about Kids' Sports Injuries

- More than 3.5 million children under the age of fourteen need medical treatment for sports injuries each year. Approximately two million high school athletes suffer sports injuries each year. Sadly, this is what keeps my medical practice in business (Powell and Foss 1999). This number does not include kids who ignore or play through their pain and injury.
- Younger children are less likely to suffer a sports-related injury or overexertion than older kids. The rate and severity of sports-related injury increases with the age of the child. This is a matter of intensity of training and increased opportunity to be injured, according to the Youth Sports Safety Alliance.

- The majority of youth sports injuries are from collisions, falls, overexertion, or being struck by something like a ball or an elbow. The most common injuries that occur during sports are sprains and strains, according to Safe Kids USA.
- Thankfully, death during participation in youth sports activities is rare. Brain injury is the leading cause of death that is sports-related. We must take concussion seriously, and I have explored the ways to lessen the "impact" of concussion in chapter 3. Some 21 percent of all traumatic brain injuries in children occur during sporting activity in the United States. (Almost half of all head injuries related to leisure sports and recreation among kids are from bicycle, skating, and skateboard accidents, says the Youth Sports Safety Alliance, with excellent tracking information). Now you know why we doctors recommend children and adults wear helmets while performing these activities.
- About half of all sports injuries to middle school and high school students are from repetitive trauma and overuse. For example, serious shoulder and elbow injuries among youth baseball and softball players have increased five times since 2000. Even children as young as eight will start to see changes in the anatomy of their shoulders in response to repetitive throwing (Mair 2007). I discuss the common injuries in chapter 3. But kids in this age group are growing, and their bones are immature. They are often not getting enough sleep or rest, and they may lack proper training and conditioning. These are all contributing factors to overuse injuries. I explain the problems here in more depth in chapter 2.
- Girls are different. The female triad can lead to serious health issues on the playing field and off. I explore the problem and the solution in chapter 4. If you have a girl who plays sports, read this chapter first.
- What is it about boys and football? I reveal my answer about whether I'd let my son play football in chapter 5.

- Certainly the more severe sports injuries are seen in contact sports such as football (Rauh et al. 2000). But in general, injuries are more common in running sports. This information comes from research my colleagues and I have conducted, and I give more information about the injury trends in chapter 2 (Feder, Frey, and Sleight 2010).
- When parents are asked about the injuries their children had sustained, it is not surprising that about 30 percent reported their child had been injured while playing a team sport. Half of the parents stated in the same survey by Safe Kids USA that the child has had more than one injury. About 25 percent of the reporting parents stated that the injury was serious. That's the role of prevention, and it's up to parents, coaches, trainers, and the athletes themselves to stay safe. I discuss ways to prevent sports injuries, in depth, in chapter 6.
- Most sports injuries (62%) occur during practices and not during games. Logically, there are more practices than games. Some of the time, the same safety precautions are not taken during practice as would be taken for a game (Safe Kids USA). Why? Parents and coaches need to take precautions with young athletes all the time. I offer my best advice to them in chapters 6 and 7.

Physiologically, children may be more at risk for injury because they are still growing, have immature skeletons, and an immature nervous system. In addition, kids today may be more aggressively athletic than ever before. It is not a surprise that the number of sports injuries has increased in number and severity.

On a brighter note—and this is the good news—half of all organized sports injuries among children can be prevented. Let's do it! The other half are caused by a perfect storm of events and are not predictable or preventable. Such is life!

1

Parents Gone Wild!

Sometimes a child's sports game brings out the best—and the worst—among the parents in the bleachers. Was the ball inside the lines? The runner safe? The goal good? That's the call for the sports official, not the onlookers. And no one knows this turf battle better than a veteran referee.

"Contrary to what you may think, we are not blind, nor are we idiots," said Garrett Felix, a United States Soccer Federation referee and former PIAA-certified sports official. "We call the games according to the rules governing their play, whether it's basketball, baseball, or soccer. And we expect the fans to be courteous, respectful, and supportive."

Otherwise, you're outta there. Many times Felix has told a parent, "Get in the car and go home."

What do out-of-control parents have to do with the subject of this book? A lot. Aggressive, loudmouthed parents can be relentless in pushing their kids on the playing field (not to mention with school work and with other extracurricular activities). Too much mom and dad on the field might mean kids push themselves to please their parents and become injured.

Not that all youth sports injuries are caused by overly aggressive parents. Not at all. But think about the deadly combination coming together in a perfect storm on a playing field. And I didn't have to look far for an extreme example.

Nothing says unsportsmanlike conduct more than the widely covered incident on May 31, 2011, right in my own "backyard."

Fox Sports reported that violence erupted at a hoop tourney. "Players attacked parents and each other when a Memorial Day youth basketball tournament erupted in violence that left one player hospitalized and another arrested on assault charges."

Police were called to San Diego's Mira Mesa High when teams from Southern California's San Fernando Valley began brawling at the end of their game, according to NBC San Diego. The tournament involved varsity, JV, and traveling teams.

"The semifinal game between the Rising Stars of San Fernando Valley and the Granada Hills Eagles had been so rough that referees ended it a minute early. Parents and spectators exchanged words and taunted players on the court, according to police on the scene, and then things got violent when a coach confronted parents who allegedly used a racial slur. A fight broke out involving at least fifteen people," a witness reported to NBC San Diego.

"Within about twenty seconds, almost the entire Eagles team ran over to the stands and started attacking one of the Rising Stars parents," according to a witness and reported by NBC San Diego.

One player had his nose broken after an Eagles player, who was arrested, allegedly punched him. The injured player was hospitalized, while the Eagles player was released from custody.

One official called the Eagles players "future criminals" and said they and their coach would be banned from the tournament for life. "I've never seen players go and attack parents of the other team," the tournament director, Rich Goldberg, said.

One father who was a witness to the brawl added his own experiences in this actual e-mail circulated to other parents after the game: "Oh now, now … Can't we just let boys, be boys? There's no end to the emasculation of our culture and society. Isn't brawling a rite of passage for young men? It was when I was a high school kid."

If you think this is an isolated problem, you are incorrect. A quick Google search uncovered nearly five million "hits" on the search term *kids, sports, bad behavior, kids sports*. And another four million hits on *bad behavior, adults, parents sports.*

Sports official Felix said that refs have the ultimate power to eject parents for yelling obscene language at anyone, including officials, coaches, or players on the other team. Most of the time when he is officiating, he tries to ignore the abusive comments being hurled at him until the heckler steps over the line.

"When the comments start interfering with the progress of the game," he said, "when the fun is taken away and other fans are feeling uncomfortable, then I step in and tell the rude fan to get in the car and go home."

The game doesn't continue until the offender has left. Certain unprintable phrases are cause for immediate ejection from the venue, with no second chances. Brawling, hitting, and shoving are way over the line, of course. Then the police get to sort things out.

"The game is for the enjoyment of the young kids," Felix said. "Yelling hurtful things doesn't change the outcome of the game or help anyone."

You're Outta Line

The vice-president of a Central California Little League district was asked to comment on bad behavior that she might have noticed on the part of parents. Her response in a personal communication to me was this:

"Let me think. Do drunk parents count? It's mostly bad behavior to umpires, which is really a no-no until you get to high school. Then it is encouraged, and parents all yell at the umpires. I think parents (mom and dad—I've seen it both) coaching from the stands are the absolute worst; embarrasses the kid, disrespects the coach, and makes dads look like jerks."

GREAT EXPECTATIONS

It has become more common recently to see parents with out-of-control behavior at kids' sports events. Sure, parents feel some emotional stress watching their children play sports, and the pressure only increases as the kid moves into more competitive and elite levels of play. Part of the problem is the parents themselves, but part is a result of how team sports are organized and orchestrated.

Parents may be guilty of building their own egos through their kids' sports. Parents are excited when their child wins. Seeing the child lose can be a letdown, and strong negative feelings appear—no matter how hard a parent might try to mask them. When parents feel elation when their child wins, be prepared for the opposite, negative emotion when they lose. This has been referred to as winning and losing by proxy.

For dads, the male hormone testosterone may magnify the positive effect of winning and the negative effect of losing. Testosterone has a lot of roles—some good, some perhaps counterproductive. New research reported in *Scientific American* suggests that testosterone can make people more poised for aggression, even if they're not feeling feisty (Mims 2007).

It has been noted that men have a greater feeling of euphoria than women when their child wins. Women are thought to get a small boost from winning but feel almost as good about when their kids are playing well.

Men desire a win more than women to maintain an emotional high, and this craving can bring out some very bad behavior. Any behavior is often justified to avoid losing, which is associated with an extreme emotional letdown. Dads in this situation don't consider how their children feel (which is extreme embarrassment in many cases). The win is all about feeding the dad's ego.

Let's not overlook the idea that dads, especially, may be reliving their glory days on the pitching mound or gridiron through their children's participation in sports. If dad was a campus hero or a high school star, he has certain expectations for his kids. If he wasn't anywhere near great, his pressure on his children to fulfill his (not their) dreams may be even greater.

Think about the motivation this dad must have had. During a high school basketball game, I observed one player stop in the middle of the game. He stood at midcourt, turned to face his father in the stands, and yelled, "Shut up."

A small round of applause resounded as the father, after coaching his son from the stands while screaming for half an hour, shrank into his seat. I don't recommend children do exactly this, but this incident tells you something about the way the young athlete felt.

In a survey of fifty injured student athletes who visited our office in the last few months, 28 percent stated that they experienced their parents, or someone else's parents, behaving badly at a game. One student commented that he sees it "all the time … I feel embarrassed for their kids." Or "My parents almost fight. I felt that it was stupid."

Other comments include, "Other parents have gotten really overenthusiastic and yelled and screamed. I just ignore everyone in the stands for the most part, good or bad." Parents can learn from their kids' reaction to the bad behavior when the kids say, "They yell and scream at the referee when he makes a bad call … I felt that parents need to set an example for us so we don't yell at the referee." But, as a player states, "Sometimes they get angry at their kids when they don't do well. I feel bad for them [the kids]."

Others commented: "Dad screams at the refs. I don't really care." Another stated that although his parents behave badly at the games, the player "felt fine because it's all out of a competitive nature." One poor kid just wants his parents to be there: "I didn't care [about parents yelling]. My parents rarely ever come to my games. They are always busy."

A few of the kids who stated they did not experience parents behaving badly commented that the parents were not allowed at games and practices. I do not know if this was school policy or the kids just didn't invite the parents.

The competition on the field or court or pool or rink may even transfer to competition with other players' parents (even parents of teammates). How well your child does may become a direct reflection of your gene pool and child rearing and the subject of ridicule and disparagement.

I have been at more than one basketball or volleyball game where a large part of the conversation among parents sitting together in the bleachers or talking in the hallways or sidelines was about how tall the player's mother and father are, and even how tall their grandparents were. Of course, this information can be put into an equation, to predict future height (see the sidebar for online calculators to predict your children's future height).

How Tall Will My Child Be?

Obviously tall parents generally create tall kids. Simple genetics. Although predicting your child's future height is not an exact science, some people like to tinker with online calculators, so here are a few:

From About.com, Pediatrics:
http://pediatrics.about.com/cs/usefultools/l/bl_htcalc.htm

From Keep Kids Healthy:
http://www.keepkidshealthy.com/welcome/yahtpredictor.html

I've overheard conversations about signs of puberty the child is showing, referring to height or hair growth. Or about a recent growth spurt. Even shoe size becomes a bragging point (the bigger the foot, the bigger the eventual kid size, in theory, and the better the basketball player—not really).

During a club volleyball game, one parent told me about Clive, who is five feet four and playing back row, but he has no hair under his armpits, she explained. The implication being that he has not even started significant puberty and, therefore, great height gains are expected.

Should we all go home and ask our sons to raise their arms and check their armpits? (Refer to the Tanner Stages in another section of this book, which explains growth in more detail.) With girls, the discussion quickly goes to whether their periods have started. This is the single biggest indicator for girls that puberty has started and advanced, although there are certain hair growth patterns that give indications of advancing puberty.

These conversations can be emotionally draining for some parents whose kids just might not "measure up," which brings me to the next point, that there are as many emotional ups and downs for the parents as there are for the young athletes.

WINNING OR LOSING: IT'S ALL ABOUT LIFE LESSONS

Playing sports is an emotional experience for kids. It builds character. Winning and losing teaches kids about the joy and disappointment in life.

The parents of athletes should have good coping skills to handle this emotional roller coaster of kids' sports. They need to be good role models for their children. But some parents just can't handle it! They experience the stress and exhibit bad behavior in many cases, such as yelling at the refs, yelling at the kids, calling the coaches and refs names, drinking alcohol at the games, and fighting with other parents. I've seen parents just storm out of a game (or not show up at all) because it is too "stressful" to watch. Seriously? This is your kid.

By the way, the parents also need to have good coping skills for the long hours, early wake-ups, long drives to games and practice and tournaments, and endless breaks in play at large tournaments and meets. Add to this the stress of the financial costs of club and high school sports. No wonder the pressure is turned up—both on the court and off.

Not every parent has the skills to cope with the bumpy ride that is involved in youth sports. Parents must be able to handle the ups and downs and also to set an example and help the kids cope.

The stress of sign-ups, deadlines, team selection (especially all-stars), equipment purchase, lineups, starting positions, playing time, advancement, private training and trainers, and finally wins and losses will elevate to such a level in some parents that they begin to behave inappropriately. The level of emotional intensity for the parents and the kids is increased as competition and specialization increase. This is a prescription for a parental meltdown in many cases.

PROTECTING THE INVESTMENT

Every investment should be protected and watched closely. Investing in your children is no different. Or is it? In youth sports, the investment is time and money and emotion on the part of parents.

Giving up time and money is considered a sacrifice. The amount of money and time required to play sports is usually large and can be a hardship for many parents. Sports can bring the kids status in their group of friends, at school, and could even make them famous (and fame comes to the parents by proxy).

Sports can get your kid into a top-notch college with a big fat scholarship and, therefore, set your kid up for a better education, job, and life. Sports can make your child a success! The pressure is on, and parents' great expectations only add to that pressure on their children.

There is so much invested—and therefore so much to lose if a child becomes injured—that pressure builds and can result in the parents behaving badly. Add to this the contact with an intense sport like hockey, basketball, rugby, or football—with the fear and risk of injury—and the intensity of the parental involvement can escalate. No question about it. These are aggressive sports to start with. There is in-your-face contact. Bravado is just part of the culture of these sports.

On a tragic note, there have been homicides in some sports such as cheerleading. You may recall the case of the mother who plotted to kill another girl's mom. Their daughters were competing for a spot on the cheer squad. The "parents gone wild" mom wanted to assure her daughter a spot on the cheerleading team, so she asked her ex-brother-in-law to hire a hit man to kill the other girl's mom, thinking the girl would be so distraught by her mother's death she'd drop off the team.

Luckily, the ex-brother-in-law brought in the police. This is extreme, but it shows the extent of the fanaticism parents may exhibit when it comes to their children's success in sports.

Think about this: You don't see a parent jumping up in a concert hall yelling at a child who misses a note during a piano recital. Or a parent throwing something at the stage when a budding ballerina stumbles. But these same parents will scream unprintable, abusive expletives that would make a football coach blush if the same kid misses a catch during a play-off game.

Dr. Brenda Bredemeier, a sports psychologist at the University of Notre Dame and co-director of the Mendelson Center for Sports, Character and Community, has reported that, during sports, normal moral reasoning is set aside and a thought process known as "game reasoning" switches on (Light Shields, Light Bredemeier et al. 2005).

This faulty thinking or game reasoning leads to parents accepting unethical and unsportsmanlike behavior because the event on the field is a sport—not real life. As if, like the breast-baring college coeds who flash the TV reality show cameras during spring break because it's not really "real," the same type of "parents gone wild" behavior is somehow okay. During the sporting event, these parents become unhinged and less civilized.

You know who they are. These are your neighbors and the parents of your kids' teammates and friends. You see them at the grocery store and in church. Maybe you carpool together or serve on the PTA. Some may be your scout leaders or coworkers. What is it about sports that brings out the beast in some parents?

TYPE A CONTROL FREAKS

Parents who are themselves type A—controlling, competitive, ambitious, and successful—are naturally attracted to youth sports. They're the pushy parents hovering like helicopters over their children. If they do it on the sporting field, chances are they're doing it over homework and household chores and paper routes and trumpet practice too.

In theory, control should be given up to the coach and officials the moment you walk into the sports arena. The bad behavior may be a result of the anxiety of giving up control to the coaches, referees, umpires, and commissioners (most of them volunteers) and trying to control events from the stands.

There are structural problems in kids' sports that a parent cannot control, and giving up control can lead to parents' frustration, anxiety, and acting-out behaviors. With age group sports, most kids get a chance "at bat." Even then a coach may not remember the minimum playing time rules, which can upset a parent.

But once a kid is playing in club sports—middle school and above—the coach will play whoever he or she needs to play to win. Some kids simply will not get off the bench. Sometimes this is not fair. This is frustrating to watch if it is your kid who's eager to get in the game but never gets a shot.

My solution? Coaches should address playing time with parents before the season starts, which, I hope, might avoid conflicts. But sports, like life, is not always fair. As a general rule, if you can score, you will play.

WHAT PARENTS SAY ABOUT WILD PARENTS

I asked some of the fathers on the AAU basketball team what they thought about the fight I mentioned earlier. Here are some snippets from three personal e-mails to me:

> Seriously, I guess we're actually now getting to that wonderful age when violence and manhood can get confused, especially when parenting is an issue and even sometimes when it's not. As a junior in high school, I had to fight my way out of a gang incident after a football game and Catholic school dance where some "punkie" public school guys showed up looking for girls and trouble. I'm sure I looked like an easy target, just like our kids do on the basketball court. I felt lucky to get some backup and escape the melee with only a gash on my forehead from brass knuckles, and the kid that hit me ended up under a parked car.
>
> Today, the stakes are a lot higher because kids didn't have guns when the violence broke out when I was a high school kid, even though I was threatened with a gun supposedly in some "gangbanger's" trench coat pocket. Regardless, it's probably

best from here going forward that our kids do all of their talking with their skill and not with their mouths.

[caps in original e-mail] *LET ME TELL YOU ABOUT THE COACHES FROM THAT TEAM! THEY DROPPED THE F-BOMB ON THEIR PLAYERS ON THE BENCH SO MUCH DURING THEIR PREVIOUS GAME ON SUN I WAS SHOCKED! THESE ARE KIDS. IT'S NOT THE NBA. SO IF THEY SEE THEIR COACHES ACTING LIKE THIS THEY THINK THAT IT'S OK TO BE AGGRESSIVE IN A NEGATIVE WAY! THOSE COACHES NEED TO WISE UP TO A NEW WAY OF TALKIN TO THEIR KIDS. THIS WAY AIN'T WORKIN! PROOF BE TOLD THEY GOT VIOLENT . . . SORE LOSERS!*

REMEMBER WHO WEARS THE WHISTLES

It may be a good idea to have parents' codes of conduct. At the very least it points out the main problem with bad conduct in youth sport: the adults. Of course, some people just need to be taught proper behavior and how to act! A code of conduct may help set some limits.

MY MEDICAL ADVICE

You can (and should) be a model spectator parent. Here's my best advice:

- **Be there.** Let your child know you support him or her by attending the games as much as you can.
- **Root for your team.** Applaud good play—no matter whose side it's on.
- **Let the coaches coach.** And let the officials call the game as they see it, not you. Remember who wears the whistles. If you go wild, you'll be sent home, and your kids will be embarrassed.
- **Let the kids be kids,** to have fun and compete.

- **Support your child athlete** because he or she will need to develop mental toughness.
- **Praise your child** for the great catch in the third inning, not the dropped ball in the bottom of the ninth. They'll learn from both experiences.
- **Educate.** If there is some knowledge you have about the sport, it is okay to review a play, even a bad play, to make it a teaching moment. None of the kids in our survey thought that yelling from the stands was a teachable moment. Most were embarrassed for themselves, the parents, and other players.
- **Remember,** many of the coaches and refs are volunteers, or receive low pay, and should be praised for being there.

2

Lumps, Bumps, and Bruises: The Risks for Kids Who Play Sports

All sports have the potential for causing injury. Heck, our kids take plenty of lumps and bumps at home and school too. They're clumsy. They stumble. They fall off bikes and skateboards and out of trees. Kids swing from monkey bars and bang their heads on playground equipment. They're daring, and they're the cause for plenty of parents to develop fear about injury.

Children's bones break, and broken arms and legs keep us orthopedic surgeons in business.

Now add to that the trauma and extra risk in watching our children playing a risky sport—any sport—and it's no wonder we parents see our hair turning gray (or falling out) prematurely.

Being a parent is hard work, yet it's the greatest joy on earth. But nothing is worse than when your child is running a fever, complaining about a stomachache, or comes limping off the field of play.

Kids get injured playing sports. They just do. There are many ways to get injured in sports. Whether from the trauma of collision with other players, blocking, jumping, running, being hit by a ball or object, or from overuse or poor mechanics, kids sustain injuries adults might not in the same circumstances. Sometimes it is just the perfect storm of a badly placed step, wet floor, another player's foot, or fatigue. Any sport carries the potential for causing injury.

This chapter looks at the risk factors, the sports with the greatest number of injuries, the reasons why kids get hurt in various sports in various ways, and how their bodies react to injury. If you weren't worried before, you may worry now, but at least you'll know what to worry about—and when to rely on us doctors.

THE BIGGEST RISKS FOR KIDS PLAYING SPORTS

Let's just look at the reality of the world of sports for kids. This is what we know:

- Children have less coordination, slower reaction times, immature muscularity, immature nervous systems, less motor skill, and are not as accurate as adults. By this I mean, children do not have a fully developed nervous system to control their movements and coordination. In addition, the most important part of the nervous system is the brain, and in children it is not fully mature in the areas of reasoning, emotions, and decision making. With respect to sports, this can lead to risky behavior.

- Kids are trying to develop athletic skills with immature bodies that at times cannot keep up with the demands and competitive nature of the sport. For example, it's unrealistic to expect a ten-year-old basketball player to slam dunk or for an eleven-year-old football player to run forty yards in 4.8 seconds.

- There is an increase in intensity and physical demands as the kid moves from youth to club sports and from middle school to high school. In boys, for example, the transition from tenth to eleventh grade is sometimes referred to as the "boys to men" summer because many boys go through their major growth spurt around the age of sixteen. It is not uncommon to have the team come back to school after summer break and not recognize 50 percent of the squad, as they have grown taller, voices have changed, and facial hair has made an appearance.

- Children are not mature enough to assess the risks involved with sports and often will take more risks. I have seen kids play through the pain of a broken ankle and not tell their parents. In addition, a child will feel fatigue and not report it to a coach, and then attempt a dangerous tumbling move in gymnastics. The legs wobble and the ankle rolls on the landing. There are kids who are so strongly identified as an athlete, and the presumed toughness that goes along with that designation, that they are willing to play through the pain.

- Kids are at greater risk of a sports-related injury when they first start a sport. This seems obvious, but they are being asked to do moves and maneuvers they may not have done before (or done much, without practice). Their enthusiasm may outweigh their skills.
- Girls and boys between five and nine are pretty similar in the way they move and play sports. As they mature, their body and their mechanics change. Testosterone tends to be much less in girls, especially as kids enter puberty. Testosterone is linked to aggression and aggressive play. At a certain point, boys are just more aggressive than girls, due to hormonal differences.
- In addition, once they get older, and the body changes, girls tend to develop differences in mechanics compared to boys. For example, wider hips in girls cause the knees to move more to the center of the body (knock-knee pattern) during the landing, as the body tries to balance itself. Studies have shown that girls, as they get older, start to land from a jump with their knees moving inward (knock-knee), which can put their ligaments at risk for injury. When they are younger, they tend to move and land from jumps more like boys.
- Society encourages boys to be more aggressive than girls. This may be changing on the sports field, but in the end, nature and hormones rule. The 1972 federal law, Title IX, mandated that there be equal opportunity in sports for girls and boys. This has resulted in a couple of generations of girls who believe they are just as tough as the boys. They are the warrior girls with deserved and equal opportunity on the field. But, in the end, estrogen rules the day. Higher levels of testosterone in boys allow them to add more muscle and get stronger than girls,

without much effort. Girls start to add more estrogen as they go through puberty, which promotes the retention and production of fat. Estrogen also makes the ligaments of girls more flexible and lax. More muscle must be added to stabilize the female joints. This is a risk factor for injuries, such as ligament tears in the knee.

- During puberty (about ages ten to fourteen) boys report more injuries (rate and severity) than girls because they are bigger, stronger, and the hits are heavier on the playing field. In addition, boys now have more testosterone and are developing mature muscles. They simply can hit harder because they are more physically mature than before. But there is another factor as well: record keeping. When it comes to the absolute numbers, boys have more injuries than girls. But football is thrown in with those numbers for boys, and when actual sports are compared that both boys and girls play (such as soccer, basketball, and volleyball), the numbers seem to be equal and in some cases higher for girls. Furthermore, the injury data for high schools is collected in a way that ignores many injuries. High reported injury rates for boys are based on ER visits, which tend to be fractures, major lacerations, and ligament tears. Yet many kids go to trainers, family doctors, and pediatricians for injury treatment. These injuries may not be reported. There are also the kids who just play through an injury.

- New data from Ohio State University and Nationwide Children's Hospital in Columbus, Ohio, indicate that girls may be more prone to ankle sprains, hip pain, and back pain. They are more likely to have chronic knee pain. Furthermore, in sports that both sexes play, such as soccer and basketball, girls may actually suffer more concussions. The reports indicate that female high school basketball players may have three times the concussion rate as the boys, and in soccer they had one and a half times the rate. The NCAA statistics suggest that female soccer players have the same rate of concussions as football players (Marar et al. 2012).

- Between the ages of ten and fourteen, boys are twice as likely to be treated in a hospital emergency room for a sports-related injury than girls. In addition, boys more often suffer from multiple injuries than girls.

- The risk of a sports injury is associated more with a child's developmental stage than with the child's chronological age or body size. Given the same age and weight, a child who is developmentally mature is at less risk for injury than an immature kid because the immature child has open growth plates, less developed muscularity, and a less developed neuromuscular system in general. Muscles protect joints and give the child strength against an opponent. Open growth plates are a common area for injury in the growing kid. The neuromuscular system contributes to balance, coordination, and ability to resist the blow from a contact sport or the awkward landing from a jumping sport. A more mature athlete can run faster, jump higher, land solid, hit harder, throw farther, and play smart.

- Developmental maturity can be graded with the Tanner Stages (see the examples later in this chapter). The speed of development toward maturity is determined for the most part by genetics and not by all the Wheaties and protein shakes they are devouring (Marshall and Tanner 1969, 1970).

- The risk of sports-related injury is dependent not only on use of protective gear but also on the condition of the playing surface. Poorly fitting equipment and badly maintained playing surfaces can cause injuries. Fields, floors, and mats should be maintained. For example, a slippery gym floor has caused more than one injury to the ACL (anterior cruciate ligament in the knee) and severe ankle sprain.

- Safety rules should be developed and enforced. Adult supervision should be present for every practice and game. There should be no distractions on the field or bench, including iPods, cell phones, food, animals, parents, friends, or other interferences.

- Kids are still developing their bones and have very unique biology compared to the adult frame they will eventually grow into. The growth plate in the bones is an area where kids can get injured. Adults do not have growth plates. Our bones have matured. I explain this physiological fact later in this chapter.

If you take all this information into consideration, you can see why children are at higher risk than adults for sustaining a sports-related injury.

What Is Considered a Sports Injury?

No exact and common definition of an athletic injury exists. There are no uniform ways to measure the severity of an injury, which makes it difficult to compare one injury report to another—or even capture realistic numbers.

In the medical literature and in practice, most injuries are defined by how the injury might adversely affect the athlete's performance (in other words, did the athlete lose time playing the sport?) (McLain and Reynolds 1989). This would exclude some injuries that are serious but do not affect a kid's ability to participate. For example, a player can break his or her wrist but still play soccer. A water polo player can sprain an ankle and still participate.

Also, player position can make a difference. A baseball player can still hit but avoid running after a fracture to the great toe, for example. However, using lost time from games and practice seems to be the cleanest way of evaluating athletic injury.

When a kid gets a sports injury, he or she has to sit it out. The athlete loses playing time, condition, and confidence. And probably the hardest thing to do after an injury is regain that confidence.

WHAT DO KIDS BREAK, BRUISE, OR INJURE?

In general, the most common sports injuries in kids are sprains and strains, although more serious injuries can occur—even, sadly, death. But we are seeing an increase in the number of immature athletes with overuse injuries.

It makes sense that if more kids are playing sports, then more kids are getting injured. Although there is a system for tracking injury for NCAA sports, there is no formal record keeping for youth league and club sports. Researchers have investigated the injury rate of the high school athlete, but even with the high school student athlete, the tracking of injuries has been limited to a few school districts.

According to the NCAA's Injury Surveillance System, over a decade ago approximately half of all injuries resulted from body contact. At the high school and recreation levels, the majority of injuries were sustained during practice.

At college and professional levels, the majority of injuries occur during competition rather than during practice. There's a reason for that: At the college level, teams are made up of selected elite-level athletes. Colleges have selected out for the most physically endowed, talented athletic players. They are in general fully mature, not growing kids. Many players in college are in their twenties, so we are talking about "adults." They have full-time trainers and medical staff and can recognize problems early and treat them. The practices are run by professionals, unlike most youth sports, which are run by volunteers.

The NAIRS (National Athletic Injury Reporting System) has indicated that not only should all injuries be reported, but also that the severity of an injury should be determined by the number of days lost from play because of the injury (Zemper and Dick 2007). NAIRS describes the following categories:

1. No report of injury: no time lost.
2. Minimum injury reports one to seven days lost from play.
3. Moderate injury reports eight to twenty-one days lost from play.

4. Major injury reports more than twenty-one days lost from play.
5. Severe injury reports a permanent disability.

The federal government has been tracking sports injuries, and the most current data available are from the Consumer Product Safety Commission (CPSC at www.cpsc.gov). CPSC is the government agency that is charged with protecting the public from unreasonable risks of injury or death. You may hear from them about cribs that can pose a danger to infants or child safety seat recalls. They also track sports injuries.

The CPSC's National Electronic Injury Surveillance System gathers injury reports from emergency departments of about one hundred hospitals across the country. These are the sports and types of injuries reported from the 2006 (most current available) data.

This list is in order of most injuries to least reported, starting with basketball at over a half million in one year. Although these are injuries for all ages, they represent the most common injuries young athletes sustain in these particular sports too:

- Basketball: cut hands, sprained ankles, broken legs, eye and forehead injuries.
- Bicycling: feet caught in spokes, head injuries from falls, slipping while carrying bicycles, collisions with cars.
- Football: fractured wrists, chipped teeth, neck strains, head lacerations (cuts), dislocated hips, jammed fingers.
- ATVs, mopeds, minibikes: although not a sport for our purposes here, the injuries show how dangerous these activities are when compared with sports: thrown from vehicles, fractured wrists, dislocated hands, shoulder sprains, head cuts, and back strains.
- Baseball and softball: head injuries from bats and balls, ankle injuries from running bases or sliding into them.
- Exercise, exercise equipment: twisted ankles and cut chins from tripping on treadmills, head injuries from falling backward from exercise balls, ankle sprains from jumping rope.

- Soccer: twisted ankles or knees after falls, fractured arms during games.
- Swimming: head injuries from hitting the bottom of pools, leg injuries from accidentally falling into pools.
- Skiing and snowboarding: head injuries from falling, cut legs and faces, sprained knees or shoulders.
- Lacrosse, rugby, and other ball games: head and face injuries.

WHICH SPORTS ARE THE MOST DANGEROUS?

With that overview, let's take a look, sport by sport, at the most dangerous sports for kids.

One recent injury survey by Safe Kids USA (2009) of kids five to fourteen years of age found that among these young athletes, the injuries occurred in football (28%), baseball (25%), soccer (22%), basketball (15%), and softball (12%). These kids also account for nearly 40 percent of all sports-related injuries treated in hospital emergency departments. But remember, not all the injured ever get to the emergency room.

Among this same age group, the highest reported risk for sports-related death is in baseball. Surprisingly, three to four kids each year are reported to die from injuries that occurred while playing baseball.

The fatal injuries are almost always a result of being hit by the ball either in the head or the chest. The catcher and the pitcher are most at risk for contact with the ball. These are horrible tragedies, and all precautions should be taken to protect the kids from harm. Protective gear, a safe distance from the ball, technique, and a high level of awareness during play will help prevent these injuries.

SURPRISING RESULTS FROM MY CALIFORNIA HIGH SCHOOL STUDY

My colleagues Keith Feder, MD, and Jill Sleight, ATC (a certified athletic trainer), and I conducted a study in 2010. We reported on 7,890 injuries in student athletes from twenty-seven California high schools. Data were collected for three consecutive school years. Information was recorded on incidence and location of injury.

In our sample, 62 percent of the athletes were male and 38 percent were female. Nearly forty thousand athletes were evaluated for this study. We defined an injury as any mishap that occurred during a competitive event or practice that caused the athlete to miss one game or meet, or two or more practice sessions. The definition was expanded to include athletes who had to decrease or change their workout routines because of pain for two or more practice sessions.

The duration of the injury was recorded by coaches, athletic trainers, or the team physician. Athletes were returned to sports when they were able to compete without restrictions.

In what we call the Frey study, injuries occurred 50 percent of the time during games and 50 percent during practice. Football was responsible for 48 percent of the injuries overall. Football resulted in the highest injury rate for males. Soccer resulted in the highest injury rate for females in this study. The majority of injuries were in the lower extremity (legs, knees, ankles, feet) for both male and female athletes.

Here is what we found:

- Ankle, 1,974 injuries (25%)
- Knee, 1,052 injuries (13%)
- Wrist, 875 injuries (11%)
- Lower leg, 627 injuries (8%)
- Upper leg, 542 injuries (7%)
- Shoulder, 444 injuries (6%)
- Back, head, foot, hand, general abrasions/contusions made up the rest of the injury categories.

The sport with the most injuries, as already stated, was football (48%), followed by basketball (16%), soccer (9%), volleyball (8%), and track and field (7%). Other sports were reported on, but had less than a 5% injury rate for each sport. The rest of the sports studied included baseball, badminton, cross-country, cheerleading, golf, gymnastics, softball, swimming, tennis, water polo, wrestling, lacrosse, and surfing (remember, we're in California!).

We analyzed specific positions played for certain sports to see if that made a difference in injuries. To look at a specific position, only the injuries that occurred during a game were studied. During practice, not only do the players play their position, but they participate in strength, conditioning, and drills that do not reflect a specific position.

For example, of all the game injuries in volleyball, the outside hitter was the most commonly injured with 118 injuries, followed by middle blocker with 81, the setter with 74, and the back row with 55.

Football had the following game injury rate per position: wide receiver, 61; linebacker, 51; running back, 43; quarterback, 28; and defensive tackle, 21.

During games, baseball had 24 injuries to the pitcher, 21 at second base, 20 at catcher, 20 at shortstop, 18 at first base, 18 at third base, 14 in center field, 9 in left field, and 4 in right field.

During meets, track and field had the following injury rates: sprints, 23; shot put, 10; long jump 6; high jump, 5; and discus, 1.

Our findings about injury rates were similar to those of other researchers, who reported that football, wrestling, basketball, and track and field resulted in the highest injury rate for boys and that basketball, volleyball, softball, gymnastics, and cross-county had the highest injury rate for girls. Girls' soccer was not reported in other studies (McLain and Reynolds 1989; Garrick and Recqua 1973).

Let me describe just one recent study published in the *American Journal of Sports Medicine* from 2011. Researchers studied one hundred high schools in the United States. Eligible schools had a National Athletic Trainer's Association (NATA) certified athletic trainer (ATC) and reported and categorized injuries using a defined and consistent reporting system.

Information was collected for nine sports: boys' football, boys' and girls' soccer, girls' volleyball, boys' and girls' basketball, boys' wrestling, boys' baseball, and girls' softball. Severe injury was defined as any injury that resulted in a loss of more than twenty-one days of sports participation, as I discussed earlier. Loss of participation is really only one consistent way we can look at the severity of sports injuries (Nationwide Children's Hospital).

According to the study, severe injuries accounted for 14.9 percent of all high school sports-related injuries. After football injuries, wrestling, girls' basketball, and girls' soccer had the highest levels of injury.

This study reported that male athletes were at higher risk of injury than females, in general. Most of the injuries occurred in football, a male-dominated sport. Among directly comparable sports (soccer, basketball, and baseball/softball), girls sustained a higher severe injury rate than boys.

Regardless of the sport, if a student athlete had a severe injury it was usually to the knee (30%). Otherwise, the severe injuries were seen in the ankle (12.3%) and shoulder (10.9%). Additionally, 5% of the severe injuries recorded were a direct result of an illegal player activity, such as spear tackling or tripping. Spear tackling is considered illegal and is a tackle in which the defender tries to bring down the offensive player by leading with the head (like a spear) during the tackle.

In general, regardless of severity, ankle sprains were the most common injury reported in this study. Previous studies agree that the ankle is the most frequent site of injury resulting in at least one day off. Knee injuries were the second largest category of injury.

Ultimately, such findings should provide a database for coaches, trainers, and sports medicine doctors involved in the care and prevention of injuries for student athletes.

WHY KIDS DROP OFF A TEAM

The short answer is injuries. It has been reported that the most common reason for dropping off a sports team is an injury. In a study of 674 high school student athletes, the dropout rate from sports, overall, was 26 percent. The rate went up to 29.8 percent if the kid played more than one sport (DuRant 2007).

When kids drop off a sports team, injury has been noted to be the most common reason in general (25%), followed by being cut from the team (19%), having a job (13%), inconvenient schedule (11%), and needing more time to study (10%).

It has also been reported that for kids who drop off a team, the highest rate was seen among African-American students, injured kids in general, injured football players, and those who had a knee injury. Other reasons cited in other studies included interest in playing another sport or activity, lack of playing time, overly competitive environment, bored, stress, dislike of the coach, and not having any fun.

In general, kids who dropped out of a sports program were noted to feel less a part of the team. These kids also reported less enjoyment, less support from their fathers for participation, often thought their poor performance was from lack of ability, and often disliked their coach.

Another study that looked at the rate of dropout from sports noted that by age thirteen, 70 percent of kids drop out of youth sports. The top three reasons in this study were adults, coaches, and parents (Ewing and Sefeldt 1996).

On the other hand, it has been reported that a kid is more likely to stay in the sport if he or she has a positive coach, according to the Positive Coaching Alliance.

In my opinion, the age of thirteen is an important transition year, in general, for kids' sports. It is the year that many of the kids are entering puberty, transitioning to high school, and leaving the age groups of club and youth sports. Little League is over at twelve. At thirteen most girls are well into or have finished growing. Kids are feeling more freedom from their parents' influence once they are teenagers and are developing other interests.

High school is starting, and it is difficult to play and get on a high school team. The level of competition increases significantly once these student athletes hit the high school years. Many of the kids who drop off the sports teams may pick up drama or Model UN or other extracurricular activities, so it is not always a bad move.

A SPORT-BY-SPORT INSIDER'S GUIDE TO INJURIES

I look at the different types of injuries our kids sustain while playing sports in the next chapter, but here I take each sport, one by one, to alert parents, coaches, and trainers about the particular dangers inherent in the sport itself. And I'll offer some prevention tips from my playbook too.

Football

I'm often asked if I would let my sons play football. I do let them. But I know the risks too. Football sends over a million kids each year to doctors' offices, emergency rooms, and hospitals.

The most common injuries in football are bruises, sprains, strains and pulled muscles, tears to soft tissues such as ligaments, broken bones, internal damage (bruised or damaged organs), concussions, and back injuries. Knees and ankles are the most common sites for these injuries.

Safety is of utmost importance and includes playing with a properly fitted helmet, mouth guard, shoulder pads, athletic supporters for males, chest/rib pads, forearm and elbow and thigh pads, shin guards, proper shoes, and plenty of water.

The football organization can help prevent injury by encouraging the proper use of safety equipment, warm-up exercises, upkeep of playing surfaces, medical personnel present during games/practice, proper coaching techniques, and conditioning.

Case Study: Meet PA, age sixteen; sport: football

It was the CIF final game. "I was playing special teams, and it was at kickoff. I remember everything about the play and the injury. I took off running so fast to run around the wedge. A kid on the other team ran around at an angle. I ducked my head down and hit him in the hip. I felt like I was floating, and then I was on the ground and could not move. I was happy we had made the play."

But he goes on to say: "I could not move or talk, like someone was holding me back from talking. The ref ran on the field; I could not move, and I was praying. My father was praying, and about ten minutes later my feeling came back. I was very alert the whole time. I had my helmet on, no one took it off." (Note: That is the right thing to do. When the shoulder pads are also on, the helmet helps stabilize the neck.)

"I wanted the trainer to let me get up and let me walk it off, but he told me the paramedics were on the way. But I did not think the injury was that serious." In the ambulance, PA found it hard to breathe. When he got to the hospital, he was evaluated and told that he had suffered a severe fracture of the C-5 and C-4 vertebrae. He had broken his neck. He was told that he needed emergency surgery with rods and titanium screws and that his injury and the surgery might prevent him from ever playing again. He could not picture himself not playing football again. PA recalls one doctor who kept telling him he would not play again, and he told the doctor to "get out of my room!"

He got a second opinion from a very experienced spine surgeon, who suggested a surgery that would allow him to play again. It included the use of bone graft from a donor and a plate with four screws. Friends and family came to visit and were very supportive. PA never stopped believing that he would get better.

PA remembers the day of surgery. He was excited to have the surgery. He was put into the operating room, and it took about five seconds before he was "knocked out. I woke up five hours later with no pain and a sore throat."

Rehab took about four to five months, and, he said, "I was not sure I would come back that year. But I was getting ready." He was going to wait the entire year before heading back into the game, and he had contacted the CIF about doing a fifth year of high school and having eligibility to play football. CIF declined. CIF said that he did not need to make up classes because his classes had been "frozen at the time of the injury, and the injury was around Christmas break, so I was not missing any school."

"When I found out I was not eligible for a fifth year, I called my doctor and asked him if it was okay to play. He said, 'Go for it.' He also said, 'Keep your head up and be safe.'"

PA checked with his trainer, suited up, and came back for the "last game before playoffs." The first play, "I made a tackle, and I knew that I had nothing to worry about. I was nervous at first, but after the first play, I got the feeling back, and I kept my head up. We played Chaminade and won that game."

PA states he is a much better and smarter player now. He is more than 120 percent better than before. "Less contact, more coverage." He also wants to remind other players to not "hit with the head down … or lead with the head, keep your head up!"

Support from family, friends, teammates, and the medical team helped him through his rehab, along with believing in himself. He never gave up.

He also notes that he had received a message on Facebook from the player that he hit in the hip. His hip had broken during the play.

Baseball and Softball

Baseball and softball injuries sent over one hundred thousand children ages five to fourteen to hospital emergency rooms for sports-related injuries in one year. Baseball also has the highest fatality rate among sports for kids ages five to fourteen (Lawson et al. 2009). As I explained earlier, three to four children die from baseball injuries each year, usually from getting hit in the head or chest by errant balls.

The most common injuries, as Little League parents know, are soft tissue strains of the elbow and shoulder, impact injuries that include fractures, most commonly of the ankle, due to sliding, and being hit by a ball, sunburn, and contusions (bruises).

Baseball has some special injuries such as Little League elbow, which occurs from repetitive throwing and can result in pain and tenderness in the elbow. The ability to flex and extend the arm may be limited, but the pain typically occurs after the follow-through of the throw. In addition to pain, pitchers sometimes complain of loss of velocity or decreased endurance and distance.

Safety is improved by using a batting helmet, shin guards, elbow guards, athletic supporters for males, mouth guard, sunscreen, cleats, hat, and detachable "breakaway bases" rather than traditional, stationary ones. Proper conditioning, warm-ups, and pitch counts also improve safety.

Kids who pitch have an increased risk of shoulder and elbow injuries. Studies have reported that there is an increasing rate of injuries and surgery to the shoulder and elbow in young pitchers who are still growing and have open growth plates. This may be from poor pitching form, early introduction of the curve ball, and overuse.

Overuse is the most common problem for these injuries. It has been noted that the kids who get injured in pitching tend to pitch more innings, throw more balls, and pitch more months in a year when compared to the kids who do not get injured. Baseball's governing bodies—USA Baseball and Little League Baseball—have noted this "epidemic" and made rules to limit the number of pitches thrown in a given week (see the box for details).

Little League Baseball Rules

Pitchers league age 14 and under must adhere to the following rest requirements:

- If a player pitches 66 or more pitches in a day, four calendar days of rest must be observed.
- If a player pitches 51 to 65 pitches in a day, three calendar days of rest must be observed.
- If a player pitches 36 to 50 pitches in a day, two calendar days of rest must be observed.
- If a player pitches 21 to 35 pitches in a day, one calendar day of rest must be observed.
- If a player pitches 1 to 20 pitches in a day, no rest is required.

Pitchers league age 15 to 18 must adhere to the following rest requirements:

- If a player pitches 76 or more pitches in a day, four calendar days of rest must be observed.
- If a player pitches 61 to 75 pitches in a day, three calendar days of rest must be observed.
- If a player pitches 46 to 60 pitches in a day, two calendar days of rest must be observed.
- If a player pitches 31 to 45 pitches in a day, one calendar day of rest must be observed.
- If a player pitches 1 to 30 pitches in a day, no rest is required.

Added to the daily and weekly restrictions on young pitchers, it is also recommended that they do not pitch in competition or showcases for a minimum of four months of each year. Throwing that is not counted in a pitch count should also be limited, but is very hard to count. It is important that the young pitcher avoid excessive warm-ups and playing catcher.

If the young pitcher's elbow or shoulder is sore, the player may have an injury. It is important to report that soreness to the coach or parents. A good rule of thumb is if the adolescent pitcher requires anti-inflammatory medications, such as aspirin or ibuprofen, or needs to ice after each game, there is an injury that needs to be taken seriously and the player should rest. If the pain does not go away after a few days of rest, then the kid needs to see a doctor.

Soccer

Common soccer injuries include ankle sprains, twisted knees, fractures of the forearm and facial lacerations. To help prevent injury in soccer, the American Academy of Pediatrics recommends that players wear protective eyewear and mouth guards to reduce the number of some head and facial injuries. Further research is needed to determine if rule changes, equipment modifications, or further safety rules can reduce the number of other injuries.

Fatalities during soccer have been strongly related to head impact on goalposts. Goalposts should be set up in a manner consistent with guidelines developed by the manufacturers and the Consumer Product Safety Commission.

There is a risk for permanent cognitive impairment (brain injury) from heading the ball. However, not enough research yet supports a recommendation that young soccer players should stop heading the ball. Supervisors of youth soccer should minimize the use of heading the ball until the risk for permanent brain damage is studied fully.

Parents, coaches, and soccer groups should work to enforce all safety rules, regulate against aggressive behavior, and strongly promote sportsmanship.

Track and Field

Common injuries in track and field include strains, sprains, and scrapes from falls. Also common are shin splints. Shin splints cause pain and discomfort on the front of the lower parts of the legs (shins). Shin splints are often caused by repeated running on a hard surface or overtraining at the beginning of a season.

Safety can be improved if participants in track and field events would wear proper shoes, athletic supporters for males, and sunscreen. It's essential for athletes to drink plenty of water. Injury can be prevented in many cases with proper conditioning and coaching.

Basketball

Basketball is now one of the most popular sports for young people in the world. However, it is also one of the highest contributors to sports and recreation injuries. An estimated 574,000 injuries involve children ages five to fourteen each year.

The overall injury rate is slightly higher for females than for males, with females having more severe injuries and more injuries requiring surgery. The most common surgery is a repair of the ACL in the knee. Overall, the majority of basketball injuries are sprains and strains.

One Canadian study noted that more ten- to nineteen-year-olds were injured playing basketball than in any other sport or recreational activity. One in seven of all sports and recreation injuries to this age group occurs while playing basketball.

According to a study of high school basketball players by the National Athletic Trainers Association (NATA), 22 percent of all male basketball players sustained at least one time-loss injury each year. Approximately 42 percent of the injuries were to the ankle/foot—far outnumbering other injured body categories such as hip/thigh (11%) and knee (9%).

Overall, sprains were the most common type of injury (43%). General trauma was the second most common type of injury (22%). Sixty percent of the injuries occurred during practice. Fifty-nine percent of game-related injuries occurred during the second half of the game.

For elementary children in physical education class, 20 percent of injuries are from basketball. Their injuries usually affect the arm (over 55%), because of underdeveloped motor skills and limited technique for catching a ball. As kids age and improve their ball-handling technique, injuries to the legs are more frequent.

At the high school level, one of every four basketball players, both male and female, have been reported to suffer at least one injury per year that results in time lost from play or practice. Males fifteen to nineteen have the highest injury rate for boys who play. Females ten to fourteen are the most frequently injured age group for girls who play. All players in all positions are at risk of suffering injuries.

In high school, the majority of injuries in basketball are to the legs, ankles, and knees. The most frequent injury is an ankle sprain (over 40% of all injuries), followed by knee injuries, wrist/hand injuries, and jammed fingers. Ankle and knee injuries, along with calf injuries, are the most severe and result in the most loss of playing time.

The most common injuries include sprains, strains, bruises, fractures, scrapes, dislocations, cuts, and injuries to teeth, ankles, and knees. Injury rates are higher in girls, especially for the anterior cruciate ligament or ACL (the wide ligament that limits rotation and forward movement of the tibia at the knee).

Pain in the front (anterior) part of the knee is common in youth basketball. Anterior knee pain is pain in the front of the knee under the kneecap. The knee can be sore and swollen due to tendon or cartilage inflammation.

The cause is usually muscle tightness in the hamstrings or quadriceps, the major muscle groups around the thigh that insert around the knee. There is also a growth plate in this area, which can lead to knee pain if inflamed and with overuse. The condition is called jumper's knee. In the next section, I explain the importance of growth plates in children and why their injuries can affect these growth plates. Spoiler alert: adults don't have growth plates. You're already fully grown.

Basketball safety can be improved with the use of eye protection, elbow and knee pads, mouth guards, athletic supporters for males, and proper shoes. Drinking water is also a safety issue to keep tissues hydrated.

If playing outdoors, players should wear the appropriate shoes because indoor shoes wear down quickly on the outside courts.

Injuries can be prevented in many cases with a program of strength training (particularly for knees and shoulders), aerobics (exercises that develop the strength and endurance of heart and lungs), core strengthening, warm-up exercises, proper coaching, and use of safety equipment.

Off-season training and good nutrition can also play a role in injury prevention. More about this in chapter 6.

Gymnastics

Thousands of gymnastics injuries occur each year. The most common injuries in gymnastics are sprains and strains of soft tissues. Safety can be improved with the use of athletic supporters for males, safety harnesses, and joint supports (such as lightweight braces and tape).

As in every sport, being properly hydrated with water is essential. Coaches should be reminding their athletes to drink water at appropriate times and amounts.

Cheerleading

Cheerleading has about four hundred thousand high school participants, and almost all of them are female.

Twenty-nine states recognize cheerleading or "cheer" as a sport. At this time, the NCAA does not consider cheer a sport and, therefore, does not track the injuries. Despite getting no respect among sports circles, cheer includes difficult tumbling, balance, stunts, aerial work, and workout schedules as intense as any other sport.

The activity must have competition to be considered a sport. Most cheerleading is done on the sideline, hence the debate. Most pediatricians believe that cheerleading should be treated like a sport. The American Academy of Pediatrics recommended in late 2012 that cheerleading be designated a sport in high school and college. This recognition would put cheerleading under the same rules and regulations as other sports-governing bodies such as the NCAA.

No matter its status, the breathtaking stunts performed in cheerleading were the cause of tens of thousands of injuries in reported statistics, and the CPSC estimated that there were sixteen thousand emergency room visits as a result of cheerleading injuries. This may be a smaller number of injuries than seen in other sports, but it makes up 68 percent of the catastrophic injuries seen in young female athletes.

The *Wall Street Journal* (Oct. 22, 2012) reported that researchers at the University of North Carolina's National Center for Catastrophic Sport Injury Research found that 65 percent of the 128 direct catastrophic injuries to high school girls as recently as 2011 were received while cheerleading (Hobson 2012).

The injuries are typically to the shoulders, wrists, head, neck, and ankles. The most risky stunts, such as pyramids and gymnastics/tumbling, should not be done on hard ground and surfaces—yet they often are. Although, a spokesperson from the American Association of Cheerleading Coaches and Administrators notes that the use of a thick mat during the performance of a pyramid could lead to increased injuries because it is an unstable surface.

The coach and trainer should be trained in the recognition of head injuries, just like the football coach is. Cheerleaders with signs of head injury should leave the competition or game immediately.

It has been recommended that the pyramid should be limited to two body lengths high in high school and increase to 2.5 body lengths in college (for more details, see the website of the American Association of Cheerleading Coaches and Administrators). The base cheerleader must be in direct contact with the surface and remain stationary. The suspension person is more at risk when inverted or rotated on dismount, and this maneuver should be avoided.

A basket toss (the cheerleader, flyer, is tossed into the air) should not have more than four throwers. The flyer needs to keep her head above a horizontal line from the torso. One thrower must remain behind the flyer at all times.

Cheerleaders should be properly supervised at all times. They should focus on all safety requirements, including developing core strength and flexibility.

Other Risky Sports for Kids

Other types of sports and recreational activities can cause serious injury. Let's look at some of the most popular.

Sledding causes more than fifteen thousand injuries to children ages five to fourteen who seek treatment each year in hospital ERs. Obvious fixes for sledding accidents are for kids to wear helmets, not sled near trees or other obstructions, and not to pile on with bigger kids.

Snow skiing/snowboarding accidents send more than thirty-five thousand children to ERs each year. Again, helmets should be worn. Snow enthusiasts shouldn't overestimate their abilities on various slopes.

Skateboarding can scare the hell out of any parent who watches YouTube videos of risky moves by other people's kids down stairs and railings and over curbs and concrete barriers. This risky sport that just screams "danger" sends more than sixty-one thousand kids to hospitals each year. The half-pipe and street skating offer no protection if skaters aren't wearing helmets and elbow and knee pads and using common sense. Add in-line skating to this risk category as well.

I commonly see foot and ankle injuries in skateboarders. It is easy to land with their foot in an "off-balance" position and tear the ligaments of the ankle or compress the cartilage of the ankle. The injury can occur on the inside or the outside of the ankle with skateboarding.

Note: My medical group has been designated the official team doctors for skateboarding's (and other extreme sports) "Dew Tour."

Trampolines are simply danger waiting to happen. That's why owners are, in some states, required to keep trampolines behind locked gates. Nearly eighty thousand children ages fourteen and under were treated in hospital emergency rooms for trampoline-related injuries in 2008. Instruction is needed to jump safely, along with spotters and adult supervision.

Interestingly, the "bounce houses" so captivating for little kids' birthday parties and store grand openings, which look trampoline-like inside, pose great danger to little children. A child goes to the ER every forty-five seconds because of bouncing injuries.

Researchers at Nationwide Children's Hospital (Thompson et al. 2012) say inflatable bouncers are the cause of a fifteenfold increase in injuries to kids—mostly broken bones, strains, and sprains but also head and neck injuries.

Injury patterns for inflatable bouncers are similar to those we docs see on trampolines, which have national safety guidelines. Bounce houses have no guidelines. So set your own rules.

Consider the risks before allowing your children to use an inflatable bouncer. If you allow your child to use an inflatable bouncer, limit use to children six years of age and older. Make sure an adult is there to supervise while the bouncer is in use and allow only one child on the bouncer at a time. If more than one child will be on the bouncer at the same time, the children should be about the same age and size.

Ice skating injures more than ten thousand children a year. Injuries include what you'd expect, twisted ankles, injuries to the toes, twisted and sprained ankles, and fractures about the ankle.

Ice hockey, like ice skating, and its NHL equivalent can be rough. Over eighteen thousand young people under the age of eighteen were treated in ERs for ice hockey-related injuries in one year.

Boxing. Enough said. Boxing just has concussion written all over it—plus all kinds of battering and bruising. I don't care if it builds character, boxing is a risky sport. A joint statement by the Canadian and American pediatric associations warns that boxing isn't appropriate for children and teens (Purcell and LeBlanc 2011).

"In boxing, children and youth are encouraged and rewarded for hitting the head. We're saying, don't put kids in a sport where hitting the head is condoned and encouraged," said Dr. Claire LeBlanc, coauthor of the new position statement and chair of the Canadian Paediatric Society's Healthy Active Living and Sports Medicine Committee.

Apparently this opposition to boxing for kids is not new, but the evidence to support the position is so much stronger now. There is a serious danger of blows to the head and face. Yet the amateur boxing supporters feel that the sport is good exercise and requires discipline, strength, and confidence. The injury rate with boxing is actually lower than in other contact sports, such as football, wrestling, soccer, and ice hockey. But yet ...

Brain trauma is a terrible injury that can occur from repeated blows to the head. Between 1918 and 1998, 659 boxers died from a boxing-related brain injury. It is perhaps the only sport where a concussion is the most common injury that occurs. Other injuries include cuts and fractures.

Like wrestlers, boxers also must make their weight class, and children must be watched to make sure that they do not limit fluids or take water-reducing medications such as diuretics to lose weight quickly.

Volleyball. Volleyball is a big sport for boys and girls, although the number of female participants is much higher than for males. Beach volleyball has recently become an official NCAA sport for women. The most common injuries include ankle sprains, shoulder overuse injuries, back injuries (more common at the beach), and knee injuries.

Ankle sprains tend to be more common in female players, so many schools require the girls to wear ankle braces (more require the girls to wear them than the boys). The players at the net tend to suffer more ankle sprains, especially with the small radius of play that is common at the net.

BODY PARTS AND GROWTH PATTERNS YOU NEED TO KNOW ABOUT

Young athletes are either still growing or have only recently reached skeletal maturation. On average, females obtain their full height at age fourteen, and males at age sixteen. However, there is a wide range of skeletal maturation rates, and variations of a year or two on either side of the averages is not unusual.

The so-called adolescent growth spurt typically begins about two years before skeletal maturity and peaks during the following twelve months, and then gradually slows to a stop during the twelve months prior to maturity (of the skeleton, not emotional or psychological maturity, unfortunately).

Adolescence is the peak of growth in a kid, although this is not an exact science. Some kids mature faster and earlier than others. Younger children grow more slowly, as a general rule, and play with less intensity (although this seems to be changing). This may be one of the main reasons that most kids' injuries occur during adolescence.

Growth Plates

Let me define what a growth plate is. A growth plate is an area of growing tissues at the end of a bone—such as in the arm or leg—that is present in immature children and adolescents.

Growth in the long bones (thighbone and shin, for example) occurs through the multiplication of specialized cartilage cells located in the growth plates (physis) of the long bones—the part of the bone that can grow. Many bones have growth plates at both ends.

During growth, these cartilage cells multiply and move away from their point of origin, toward the center of the bone. They are then gradually transformed from cartilage to bone, and the bone grows in length. In the last year of growth, the growth plates narrow as the rate of multiplication of the cartilage cells decreases.

As growth ends, the growth plate has narrowed to the point where the bone on either side fuses together and no more growth can occur. Growth plates are located in the knee, ankle, heel, wrist and elsewhere.

The growth plate is a source of injury for many kids. Here's why: The cartilage of the growth plate is weaker than the surrounding bone and can be fractured. Fractures to the growth plate are thought to be more common during periods of rapid growth. The adolescent growth spurt is a common time for injury to the growth plate. And just for medical purposes, we call bone breaks fractures. A fractured bone is a broken bone. The severity of the "break" also can be measured.

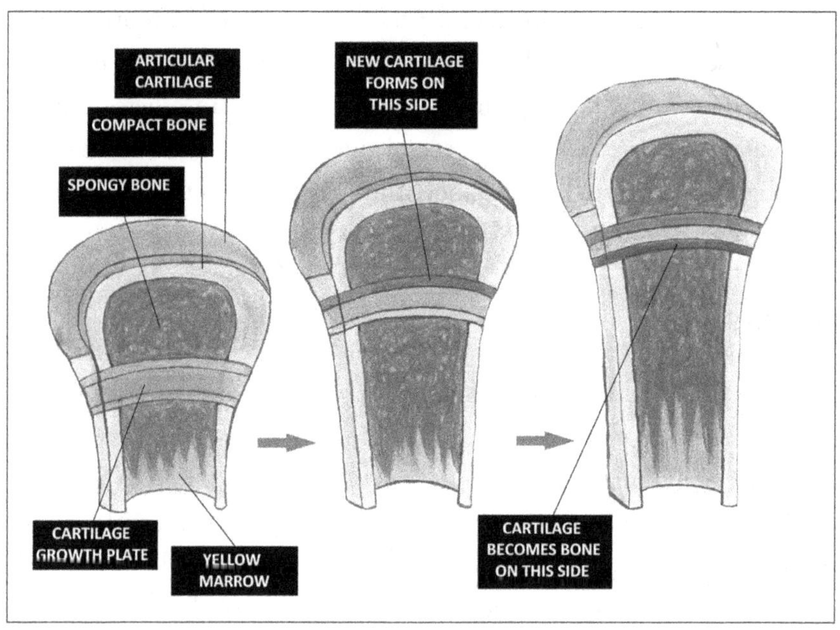

The growth plate: The growth plate is where the bone grows in children. The growth plate, also known as the physis, is the area of growing tissue at the end of the bones in kids. The growth plate determines the length and shape of the bone once growth is complete. When the bone is mature—sometime during adolescence—the growth plates are replaced by solid bone.

A hairline fracture is less serious than a bone that has been cracked open or broken in two. A compound fracture is one that has broken through the skin, which was shown on national TV during the writing of this book during the NCAA Final Four basketball playoffs. An open fracture is another way of saying compound fracture. This type of bone break is thought to be a result of more trauma and higher injury forces.

Any fracture to the growth plate is a serious injury and can result in abnormal growth of the long bone and even deformity. Although injuries of this type are hard to prevent, the consequences can be reduced if the injury is recognized and treated correctly.

An injury to the growth plate is a unique injury that only children can sustain. The growth plate can be injured with trauma or overuse. In boys, typically the growth plate is open (growing) until they are fifteen to eighteen years of age. The growth plate in girls is usually open until a year or so after she starts her periods (ages twelve to fifteen). Repetitive injuries to the growth plate are a type of stress fracture. Luckily most heal without any problem.

The most common growth plate injuries in youth sports are in the ankle and the wrist. Growth plate injuries around the ankle come as a result of a twisting injury and can produce significant swelling and severe pain with weight bearing. These injuries can be mistaken as "just a sprain." The swelling and pain with weight bearing indicate that this is a more severe injury.

Growth plate injuries at the wrist usually result from an attempt to break a fall by putting the hand out. This injury will produce swelling, pain, and even deformity around the wrist. This injury can also be mistaken as a sprain. A persistent complaint of pain, especially associated with a limp (ankle), requires immediate medical evaluation.

A special type of growth plate, the apophysis, is present at the site where many large muscles attach to bone. These growth plates have a role in shaping bones to withstand the large stress that major muscles place on them. An example of an apophysis is the back of the heel where the Achilles tendon inserts, the front of the knee at the site of attachment of the patella tendon (below the kneecap), and the medial epicondyle on the inner side of the elbow (Little League elbow) where the wrist flexors originate. These growth areas are commonly injured from overuse (too many pitches or too high a pitch count, multiple overhead spikes, or too many overhead hits and serves, depending on the sport).

Many of these overuse injuries can be prevented with proper warm-ups and stretching. Some of these injuries require a change in mechanics, such as with Little League elbow. With Little League elbow there needs to be a change in throwing mechanics, decreased use of the curve ball (among pitchers), change in position (pitcher to first base, for example), or no throwing for a while.

In general, apophyseal injuries get better with rest and will surely get worse if the painful activity is continued (or not modified). Playing through the pain will, in general, only lead to more severe pain and poor performance. Playing through pain is not character building and not a measure of toughness.

Kids Bounce Back Fast

Even though immature bones and muscles can be more at risk for injury, on a brighter note, kids recover quicker than adults.

Sometimes maturation brings a temporary decrease in balance and coordination for young athletes. During puberty, limb length, mass, and overall size all change with age. The limb length can increase 1.4 times from ages six to fourteen. The mass of the arm and leg may triple. So during growth, a mismatch in length and muscle size can lead to imbalance.

Muscles need to get stronger to move the bigger limb, and sometimes muscle strength and bone growth do not match. This creates increased strain on the tendons, ligaments, muscles, and growth plates. High-intensity sports, such as football, basketball, and lacrosse, will put all these body parts at even more risk for injury (Frank 2007).

As kids grow bigger and stronger, the risk for injury increases, largely because of the amount of force involved. For example, a collision between two eight-year-old Pee Wee football players who weigh sixty-five or seventy pounds each does not cause as much damage as that produced by two sixteen-year-old high school football players who each may weigh over two hundred pounds.

I say that but there's always the exception. It was alarming to read about a Pee Wee game in Massachusetts in September 2012 (Belson 2012). During that game between two rival teams of boys as young as ten, five had head injuries later determined to be concussions. The *New York Times* called this game "one of the more disturbing episodes in the ever more controversial world of youth football."

I agree with the sports writer who said, "Rules are only as effective as the adults charged with enforcing them." League officials suspended both coaches and barred the referees from officiating any games in that league. The presidents of the youth programs were put on probation.

Kids mature at different rates. There is often a big difference in height and weight among kids of the same age. So there was a hodgepodge of players on that Massachusetts field that day, some more mature and larger in stature than others. (And, I suspect, a lot of parents who were reluctant to say anything. Should they have? Yes.) The rough play caused serious injury to the smaller, less mature players. And the coaches and refs were also reluctant to call "mercy rules," even though the final score was 52–0.

Genetics is a big factor in how big and how fast a kid will grow. There is no predictable scientific formula to determine how big a child will eventually be, however. It helps a lot if the parents are big and tall, though.

The Tanner Stages

The Tanner Stages of classification provides a scale for following the maturity and development of a child (Marshall and Tanner 1969, 1970). The scale is based on external sex characteristics. The size of the breasts, genitalia, and growth of pubic hair are evaluated. James Tanner, a British doctor, developed the scale. The stages are different for girls and boys.

We humans pass through the Tanner Stages based on genetics and when we start puberty. Some kids pass through the stages faster than others, according to an adolescent medicine specialist, Dr. Lawrence Neinstein.

Here are some approximations on what the Tanner Stages evaluate. For actual illustrations, I direct you to the many illustrations on the Internet. I did not reprint them here because some would be too graphic for a handbook like this.

Tanner I
No pubic hair. On the average, this is around ten years old or younger.

Tanner II
There is minimal growth of light, soft pubic hair at the base of the penis and scrotum in boys and labia in girls. The average age for this stage is around ten to eleven and a half years of age.

Tanner III
The pubic hair is more thick and curly and starts to spread out to the sides. The average age for this stage is eleven and a half to thirteen years of age.

Tanner IV
The pubic hair looks like an adult's but does not grow on the insides of the legs. The average age for this stage is thirteen to fifteen years of age.

Tanner V

The pubic hair starts to grow on the insides of the thighs. The average age for this is more than fifteen years of age.

[Note: The author of the classification system himself has argued that age classification using the Tanner Stages is not accurate. Tanner stages do not match with chronological age and maturity stages and thus are not used for the estimation of age.]

MY MEDICAL ADVICE

It goes without saying, but I'll say it again, kids need proper training in developing the skills they need to play sports, whatever that sport is. The first weeks of a season should be used to develop skills and technique, rather than just "playing" the sport.

With youth sports, kids come in with different levels of knowledge about the sport. It is important for the coach to spend time going over the proper warm-ups and mechanics of the sport. This will help prevent injury and develop winning skills.

Players should wear safety equipment recommended for their sport—in both practice and in games—and the equipment must be the right fit.

Even more important than safety equipment is awareness of the dangers of the sport. Kids do get hit in the head with baseballs. It happens all the time. It happens in AA (first season of kid pitch) just as often, perhaps more often, than in high school!

- Teach your kids (coaches, this is for you) to look at the ball. Be aware of what is happening on the field and on the court.
- Teach your kids how to develop a sports IQ. The sports IQ has a lot to do with awareness of what is going on around the player and predicting what will happen next. The sports IQ requires the player to see the court and field. It requires the player to have good peripheral vision (we call these peripherals, for short). Some

of the best players in every league have a great sports IQ. If it will help your kid's team win and prevent injury, it is something worth teaching.

We doctors know why children need a sports physical. Not just a quick look in the ears and mouth and a height and weight check. We need to know what sport the child is going to play, and we need to do a proper medical evaluation. Parents must insist on a serious presports physical. Period.

Parents, players, and coaches need to all know and practice the safety rules. Children of the same maturity level physically (and not necessarily the same age) should be playing against each other.

I'll have many more tips on prevention in chapter 6. But for now, I urge you to follow this smart advice to keep your kids and everybody else's kids safe on the playing field.

3

From Head to Toe: Common Sports Injuries Kids Get

As a sports medicine doctor, I take care of injured athletes, and my colleagues and I see it all—broken bones, torn ligaments, sore shoulders, unstable elbows, twisted ankles, cuts, bruises, and really big bumps.

As the season turns to football, my medical practice adds yet another clinic day to the week—Saturday mornings—to handle the increased load of injured kids.

It is no coincidence that injuries abound as practices start in August and playing begins in September and October, in the peak of football season. Of course the other seasons bring in injuries, but when football season starts, the injury load definitely increases.

In addition to the usual injuries, we also see the bumps to the head and evaluate for concussions during the preseason, at the sidelines (as team doctor), and after this type of serious injury occurs.

The sports injuries that we see in young athletes can be put into three major categories: acute injuries, overuse injuries, and reinjuries. Unlike adults, kids can also suffer from growth plate injuries, because they have growing bones, as I explained in the previous chapter.

This chapter looks at the specific injuries kids get from head to toe while playing sports.

CONCUSSION, BROKEN BONES, AND OTHER ACUTE INJURIES

Acute injuries occur after a specific accident or incident. You may find this interesting: most acute injuries occur at the beginning of the season, at practice, in the last quarter of a game, or after returning from another injury. It makes sense. The young athlete is tired, still hurting, not conditioned enough—all situations that can lead to an increased risk of injury.

In kids, acute injuries typically involve minor bruises, sprains, strains, or injury to the growth plate. Compared to younger kids, high school athletes have more severe injuries of this type. The other types of sports injuries are overuse situations and getting reinjured, which I discuss toward the end of this chapter, too.

Acute injures are what you'd expect. These include broken bones and torn ligaments (a quick anatomy refresher here—ligaments are fibrous tissue that connect bones to other bones). The weak part of the bone in kids is the growth plate. It is not unusual to have an injury or break (fracture) at the growth plate with an injury. And with kids, it's sometimes hard to tell a suspected sprained ankle from a real break. Guessing wrong about that can leave the athlete with a weak ankle for life.

The wrong equipment and poorly maintained playing surfaces can put kids at risk for acute injuries. A lot of kids who play baseball and softball have suffered broken legs or ankles from sliding into immobile bases. Playing basketball on a poorly maintained or old slippery basketball court can lead to injuries of the ankle and the knee, as the player slides around. In football, an uneven field with holes can lead to more injuries, especially ankle sprains and knee ligament injuries.

The most severe acute injuries that occur include these:

- Eye injuries (including a scratched cornea, detached retina, and bleeding in the eye)
- Broken bones or ligament tears
- A broken skull (broken bones of the head, with or without a concussion)

- Concussion
- Spinal cord injuries

So let's start with the head and move down through the various parts of the body and look at the common acute sports injuries kids get, ask ourselves why these injuries are happening, and know what to do to prevent them and treat them—no matter what your role is on the playing field as coach, trainer, parent, or player.

HEADS UP: A CONCUSSION IS A BRAIN INJURY

Like the crazy cartoon characters who flop around in a daze with words like *$%&@#* in thought bubbles, kids can get conked on the head and can become disoriented during play or sports activities. You may have even heard a concussion described as "he got his bell rung" or "she had her lights punched out."

It's alarming when you see a pro football player lying on the turf after having his "bell rung" following a particularly hard tackle. It's especially scary when the player who is staggering off the field supported by two trainers is your son or daughter.

Concussions are a brain injury. They are serious, and they can occur in any sport.

It has been reported that fewer than 10 percent of football players say that a doctor or team trainer diagnosed them with a concussion, yet one-third say they had symptoms of dizziness, headache, blurred vision, and loss of balance after a head injury (Thurman et al. 1998; Israel and O'Brien 2012).

Over half of these kids said that they did not report the symptoms because they were afraid they would be pulled out of play. They also said they would be more likely to report a teammate's symptoms than their own. Many of these players do not recognize concussions as a problem, and they certainly don't want to miss play.

Consider this typical (and real) story:

"I was playing interleague summer football, where helmets were not allowed during passing tournaments, and I was not wearing one. This was between sophomore and junior year. I was reading a quarterback's eyes and scanning the field, and then he threw to an open receiver.

"As I was about to deflect the pass, I collided with another teammate, head to head, and I blacked out. I remember bits and pieces of walking to the sideline with one of my coaches at my side. I lay down on a bench on the sidelines, and I felt like I was confused and did not know where I was. The coach asked me what year it was, and I answered correctly. I do not recall any other questions. I remember his finger going side to side, and I moved my eyes, but not my head.

"My head began to hurt about ten to fifteen minutes later, 'inside my head.' The coach told me to 'go home if you are not feeling well.' If you are feeling queasy or nauseated, he told me to go to the ER, and don't go to sleep and check out.

"When I got home, I got in the shower and felt like I was going to vomit. I was very tired, and I remembered my coach's advice to not go to sleep. It was now that I realized that I may have a concussion. Keep in mind, I had taken an athletic trainers program at the high school, and it still took me this long to admit I may have a concussion.

"About one hour later we were in the ER. I had a headache, was nauseated, dizzy, clumsy, not completely oriented, and balance was poor. I felt like I was on a boat, and it was hard to place my feet in a balanced position. The doctor evaluated me with more questions. He asked me what happened and if I had lost consciousness. 'Yes,' I replied. No treatment was given, other than observation. It took me two weeks to return to normal. It took me three weeks to return to practice.

"I need to mention that I had a second concussion two years after the first. I was playing against Arroyo Grande High School, varsity squad, ranked first in the league. It was a close game, as they attempted a two-point conversion. I was playing cornerback, and the opposing quarterback rolled out as he pretended to throw the ball and then attempted to run into the end zone, instead of passing. Me, at five ten, 140 pounds meet up contact to contact, helmet to helmet with the opposing quarterback, who weighed in at six one and 210 pounds.

"The next thing I remember is the blackness that came over me; my next memory was a teammate's hand reaching for me and helping me up. I felt that the lights on the field looked like I was in a doctor's office. This is what struck me, was the brightness of the lights. We ran off the field, so they could resume play.

"My teammate noticed that I was not running in a straight line as I ran off the field. I sat down. I threw my helmet off, and I noticed that all my senses were heightened. Lights were brighter, sounds were louder and shrill, and I knew something was wrong. I felt way more out of it than my last concussion, my head hurt, my nose hurt (later I found out it was broken). The ATC came over and asked me who the president was, what year it was, and then he gave me three words to remember and then use them later in conversation. I answered all the questions right. The moving finger eye test was done, but my head was moving with the finger this time, instead of just the eyes moving [this may be a sign of a concussion].

"I remember looking around the field and being confused. I looked up at the scoreboard and saw that the opposing team had a bigger lead than before. My girlfriend was the student athletic trainer at the game, and noticed my nose was crooked. She advised me to go the hospital to get the nose checked out.

"I told the ER doctor that the injury happened helmet to helmet and that I had blacked out for a second. This happened right at the point of contact. I do not recall another thing until my teammate was reaching down for me. She evaluated my nose and said it was broken and that it needed to be reset, and I told her about the possible concussion and that I had one before. She orders a CT scan of my brain that night. I went in the scanner and lay on my back as the machine went round and round. It took a few minutes, but I felt separated from everyone else and normal events; I was alone. Those minutes in the CT scan, alone, time moves very slow.

"When the CT was over, I returned to the ER, and the doc said, 'Everything is clear.' She said my nose was broken but would have to be reset at another date. She gave me some instructions to stay out of physical contact for a couple weeks. I felt back to normal in two weeks. I returned to play three and a half weeks later.

"When I returned to the game, I was afraid it might happen again. It made me hesitate, where in the past I was fearless."

His mother was not present for the first concussion. For the second concussion, she recounts, "I saw my son so mismatched on the tackle (size, that is), when he got hit, his head went to the side, my first reaction was to let the trainers handle the situation. But the officials resumed play, and I watched as my son walked to the sidelines. I watched every move, but I did not know, at that time, that he had blacked out. He did look a little wobbly, and as a parent, you watch every move your child makes when he is called out of the game.

"It was a teammate who noticed the abnormal walking. It was the student athletic trainer who noticed the broken nose. The ATC checked out my son and advised us to go to the hospital after the game. We went to the hospital. I did not see any personality changes. I did notice the nose was curved to one side. So much for faceplates."

Signs of Concussion the Coach Might See

- Appears dazed or stunned
- Is confused about assignment or position
- Forgets sports plays
- Is unsure of game, score, or opponent
- Moves clumsily
- Answers questions slowly
- Loses consciousness (even briefly)
- Shows behavior or personality changes
- Can't recall events prior to hit or fall
- Can't recall events after hit or fall

Symptoms of Concussion the Athlete Might Mention to Coach or Parents

- Headache or "pressure" in head
- Nausea or vomiting
- Balance problems or dizziness
- Double or blurry vision
- Sensitivity to light
- Sensitivity to noise
- Feeling sluggish, hazy, foggy, or groggy
- Concentration or memory problems
- Confusion
- Does not "feel right"

Source: Heads Up: Concussion in Youth Sports, CDC fact sheets, www.cdc.gov/ConcussionInYouthSports

Sad to say, but 21 percent of all traumatic brain injuries in children occur during sporting activity in the United States. A significant number of former players have had ill effects from concussions suffered while playing. This has gotten a lot of coverage in the press, and for good reason (Gessel et al. 2007).

The CDC has created a helpful website called Heads Up: Concussion in Youth Sports with fact sheets for coaches, parents, and athletes. The site even includes an online training course in concussion for coaches (and parent coaches in youth sports would also benefit from this information).

It's the responsibility of the coach to recognize a possible concussion. Often a coach might be concentrating on game strategy and miss the signs. Then it's important for the athlete to step up and tell the coaches or parents about bumps and just not feeling right.

Parents have a role to play as well. If you think something "just isn't right about your child," whether on the playing field or after the game or practice, see your doctor right away.

It's your responsibility as a parent to let the coach know about any recent concussions in any sport, especially if your child competes in more than one activity. A clunk on the head in Saturday's football practice is not something the baseball coach on Sunday afternoon would know about—unless the player or parent tells the coach.

I've seen the effects of concussion show up days or weeks after the big game or a hard practice or a fluke hit by a baseball or lineman. These are not symptoms to ignore.

Who Gets Concussions?

The CDC has reported that 6 percent of the annual 2.4 million youth sports injuries seen in emergency rooms are concussions.

Among fifteen- to twenty-four-year-olds, playing in sports is the second leading cause of concussion. Motor vehicle accidents are the leading cause. So think of your child being in a serious car crash. That's the power of a concussion on the playing field.

Scientists at Ohio State and Nationwide Children's Hospital in Columbus, Ohio, reported in the *Journal of Athletic Training* that concussions made up 8.9 percent of all high school sports injuries. They reported on nine sports (boys' football, soccer, basketball, wrestling, and baseball and girls' soccer, volleyball, basketball, and softball). This number is about double the 5.5 percent reported a decade earlier (Powell and Foss 1999).

How do we account for more concussions? During this decade the rules of the games have changed little. Players may be wearing more protective gear and might be less cautious. Certainly, there is awareness, which may account for the increase in reporting. Injury tracking is more accurate than it was a decade ago.

More kids are participating in sports. I cannot find any evidence that kids are playing harder or that the game has become more violent. And while the CDC reports about three hundred thousand concussions per year, one researcher speculates that there may be ten times that number in reality (Thurman, Branche, and Sniezek 1998).

Even at that, one player is estimated to suffer a concussion in almost every American football game (regardless of how severe). Since 1997, about fifty youth football players (high school or younger) have died or sustained serious head injuries. Football players suffer the most brain injuries of any sport.

Surveys of high school players themselves produce frightening results because about half of players say they have had symptoms of concussion. Many do not report the symptoms for fear of being taken out of play or not seeming tough enough.

We can't see a concussion, at least not without imaging such as a CT scan or unless there is also a laceration or bloody bruise. The brain, nonetheless, has been bruised—inside. Knocked against the skull, even when encased in a football helmet. We have treatment for concussion, but we need to know about the event to be able to address it.

There is a critical time period after injury, referred to as the "concussion penumbra." During this time, the injured area is at risk for further injury (Giza and Hovda 2001). This is an important period where the player needs rest and observation—not to be put back into the "big" game.

Once a concussion occurs, the brain requires more nutrition, blood flow, oxygen, and rest for recovery. The brain tissue must recover or more injury may occur.

The concussion penumbra is a period of time when there is tenuous equilibrium between brain healing and the need for increased nutrition and blood flow. The timing and degree of this period differs depending on the developmental age of the brain. There actually may be more swelling in a child's brain. Within a few days, however, the brain's physiology may begin to go back to normal.

In high-risk sports—football, rugby, soccer, hockey, and basketball—a team doctor and trainer should be on high alert for a head injury.

The Zurich guidelines were developed after several important conferences in 2008 on concussion (McCrory et al. 2009). The guidelines are a simple yes/no scale. For example, did the player suffer a concussion?

Yes or no. Did the player lose consciousness? Yes or no. And so on according to a defined protocol.

Based on these guidelines, the NCAA has put together a concussion plan. If a player sustains a concussion during a game, the player does not go back into play. No matter what.

One of the best assessments of concussion risk is neck strength. A small decrease in change of head velocity will have a large effect on concussion risk. A stronger neck means less head displacement (Viano et al. 2007).

Assessing Concussion before the Season Begins

The Sport Concussion Assessment Tool 2 called the SCAT2 (more recently a SCAT3 has been developed) is used for diagnosis. The SCAT2 grades concussions in stages. The first stage includes loss of consciousness, amnesia, headache, neck pain, blurred vision, nervousness, and anxiety.

The SCAT2 or 3 is a series of yes and no questions and also simple numerical scores for signs and symptoms of concussion. For example, the athlete may be asked to recite the months of the year in reverse order, starting with a random month. In another measure, the athlete may get read a string of numbers and when the tester is done, the athlete may repeat them back in reverse order (for example, 9-1-7 would be 7-1-9).

The final part of the SCAT2 is a test for balance and coordination. Coordination can be checked by having the athlete standing heel to toe, hands on hips with eyes closed, and maintaining a stable position for twenty seconds. The number of mistakes is noted. A mistake would include opening the eyes or moving out of position. A concussion is diagnosed if the player makes five or more mistakes (errors) in twenty seconds.

If an injury occurs and is assessed as a concussion, the SCAT2 or 3 has a page that is meant to be given to the athlete and his parents and includes signs to watch during the next twenty-four to forty-eight hours. The athlete should not be left alone, and an adult needs to look for changes in behaviors mentioned in the box on signs of concussion.

Exercise or training should be started only after the athlete is clearly without symptoms—physical and mental. The final decision to return to play should be made by a doctor.

The SCAT2 is designed to be used by medical and health professionals. Preseason baseline testing can be useful for interpreting post-injury scores. It does not need to be administered by a doctor. (A SCAT3 has just come out that replaces the original SCAT and SCAT2.) Check to see which test your team uses.

It is a good idea for a player to take the SCAT2 test before the season starts. Even healthy kids make some mistakes on the test. A baseline test is helpful in case the player has a head injury during the season.

Of interest, one study reported that girls tested significantly better (higher total score) compared to the boys in a preseason test. The same study noted that players with previous concussions tested lower than players who had not had concussions.

A Pocket SCAT test can be used by the team doctor or medical personnel to check on a kid with a possible concussion. The test is a series of yes and no questions to assess the potential injury. In addition, numerical scores are assigned for important signs and symptoms of concussion. The test yields a total score and will determine if the player has a concussion—yes or no.

The diagnosis is not always clear-cut. This makes recognition and treatment a challenge. Errors should be made on the side of caution. I always advise that it's better to overdiagnose a concussion than to miss it altogether! Both the parent and the player are often afraid to report symptoms and signs, as they think the player may miss play. There is often the issue of cost of an expensive CT scan of the head or an examination by a physician. Some parents and players are simply not aware that a concussion is a serious matter.

There is another test called the IMPACT (Immediate Post-Concussion Assessment and Cognitive Testing). It is called a neurocognitive test. This test can be given in the preseason, like the SCAT2, to get a baseline. It is better to compare an injured player to his or her own baseline test after an injury. This makes the diagnosis on the field or in the locker room more accurate.

A computed tomography scan (a CT scan) of the head is recommended if the player is not doing well. A player that is not doing well should see a neurologist, who is a specialist in disorders of the nervous system, and that includes the brain. A CT scan is a highly sophisticated series of detailed x-rays.

Model Law Protects Players

Some states have recently passed laws mandating that every kid who suffers a concussion must be cleared by a qualified health professional before he or she can return to play. These laws are meant to protect kids from traumatic brain injuries.

The Lystedt Law is the model for this legislation and was passed in the state of Washington in May 2009. This law was named after a middle-school student named Zackery Lystedt, who returned to a football game with a concussion and was permanently disabled.

The legislation has these three important parts:

- Any player suspected of sustaining a concussion must be immediately removed from play and must be cleared by a qualified health professional before going back into the game.
- The law recommends concussion education for coaches, parents, and the young athlete.
- Parents are required to sign a form that states they are aware of concussions and the risks of concussions in the sport their child is playing.

Do you know your state's laws regarding concussion? Over half of states now have student athlete concussion laws in place and many have legislation pending. A helpful website that keeps up-to-date with state concussion laws for student athletes is Education Week, www.edweek.org.

Risky Sports for Causing Concussions

It is not just football that presents a risk for concussions. Any contact sport has a risk for traumatic brain injuries. Sports such as soccer and lacrosse are seeing a rise in concussions and have less protective gear than football. Boxing is still an obvious sport with high risk.

Sports with the Highest Rates of Concussions
(in order of highest occurrence)

Football
Girls' soccer
Boys' lacrosse
Girls' lacrosse
Boys' soccer
Wrestling
Girls' basketball
Softball
Boys' basketball
Field hockey
Baseball
Boys' volleyball
Girls' volleyball

I agree with the CDC on what to do if an athlete has a concussion or is suspected to have one. Here are more smart rules:

- Players, their parents, the team trainers, and all coaches should regularly review the signs and symptoms of a concussion.
- The player must be immediately removed from the game. No exceptions.
- Get a medical evaluation. The parents can take their child to their family physician or the emergency room. In severe and obvious cases, the coach calls an ambulance for immediate transport.

- If the athlete has a concussion, follow medical care advice. Getting better takes time. The brain needs to heal. The athlete is more vulnerable to a second concussion while recovering from the first one.
- Get the okay from a health care professional to return to play.
- Protect student athletes from concussion by making sure they are wearing recommended protective gear (helmets, padding, shin guards, eye and mouth guards). If equipment is going to protect the athlete, it has to be the right equipment for the game. It must be worn correctly. And the athlete must wear protective equipment every time.

THE FACE: TEETH AND JAWS, EYES AND CHEEKS

It's one thing to break a leg, but a jaw? Get teeth knocked out? Lose the sight in an eye that gets poked during play? A parent's worst nightmare. These types of injuries can be life changing and even life threatening. Prevention is always your best choice.

Facial trauma in sports is highest in soccer, basketball, squash, gymnastics, baseball, and volleyball. As opposed to injuries to the extremities that affect function, facial injuries involve cosmetic and functional considerations. The face protects the skull, the airway, the esophagus, and communication—not to mention your child's ability to smile.

Tooth and face injuries involve muscles, tendons, and bones. Dental-facial injuries can be associated with an injury to the airway or nervous system. Some of these injuries can be life threatening if they interfere with breathing, for example.

Let's look at the types of dental-facial injuries that occur in high school athletics and their treatment. I'll tell you how to manage these injuries on the playing field and how to get emergency treatment. And, of course, I'll give insight into preventing some of these injuries using state-of-the-art protective equipment.

Cuts, scrapes, bruises, and bumps to the face and mouth are common in many high school sports and even for younger athletes. Often, injury is the result of facial contact with another player, equipment, or a ball. Who hasn't gasped when a child is cracked in the head with a bat or a basketball player gets knocked to the hardwood after an elbow to the eye or mouth?

If there is a blow to the head or face that results in a cut or bruise (we doctors call them lacerations and contusions), the player should be checked for a concussion. Guidelines for concussion are discussed in depth earlier this chapter.

In the case of lacerations to the face, the use of steri-strips (butterfly bandages), skin glue, or stiches can be necessary. Suturing of a laceration, when necessary, should be done as quickly as possible by a doctor or trainer to avoid scarring as much as possible. And this type of injury would mean a trip to the ER.

Blows to the Mouth and Teeth

A variety of different types of injuries can take place affecting the teeth and mouth. The first of these is damage to the tooth without any visible damage. This often results in what we call a tooth concussion, which damages the blood vessels supplying the nerve of the tooth. The tooth may become discolored over time or the nerve in the tooth may die (that may mean a root canal procedure). The player may experience soreness or sensitivity with pressure or biting.

Emergency treatment is not necessary. The player should avoid direct pressure on the tooth. If symptoms get worse or do not improve, the player needs to see a dentist and get x-rays.

A blow to the mouth may be absorbed by a tooth or several teeth and surrounding structures without causing a fracture to the tooth. Sometimes the tooth is displaced and sometimes it fractures. A fracture of the crown or root of the tooth has various forms depending on the blow to the mouth.

A chipped tooth usually doesn't cause problems, but that tooth may be sensitive to temperature change or touch. The tooth edge may feel sharp under the tongue. A dentist can smooth the edge of the tooth to repair the chip.

Bigger chips can be reshaped to make the tooth appear whole again with bonding of a white resin material, much like that used in fillings. This requires a skilled dentist.

Severe fractures usually involve the front teeth and often result in nerve damage. This type of injury often requires root canal treatment. If there is no nerve damage, then bonding or porcelain veneers can be used to replace the damaged tooth. If the root of the tooth is injured, this can be confirmed by dental x-ray. Follow-up visits with the dentist are necessary to watch for possible infection.

And if the tooth is knocked out, completely, it might be able to survive and be placed back in the socket. Or not.

A knocked-out tooth is called an avulsion. The less time the tooth is out of the mouth, the better chance of a good result with treatment. Acting quickly can make the difference between keeping and losing the tooth. Within thirty minutes of the injury, there is a 90 percent chance of planting the tooth back into the mouth. After two hours, the chance for success drops to 5 percent. Proper handling of the tooth increases the success of putting the tooth back into the mouth.

Here's what to do: The knocked-out tooth should be rinsed off, but not scrubbed, to remove any dirt or foreign debris. Sterile water is preferred but you can use milk to rinse with. The tooth should then be gently wrapped in gauze and placed in Hank's Save-A-Tooth solution (if you happen to be really lucky and have this on the field in the first aid kit) or a container of milk and transported to the dental office as quickly as possible. [Note to self: Ask the coach to have this solution in the on-field first aid kit. Also, program your smartphone with your dentist's emergency number or the location of an emergency dental office in your area.]

The faster the dentist can plant the tooth back into your kid's mouth, the better. The tooth will then be splinted and stabilized for seven to fourteen days. The dentist will prescribe antibiotics to be started the day of the injury.

Cracks to the Face

The bones in the face most prone to injury in young athletes are the upper jaw (maxilla), cheek bones (zygomatic arches), the bones that form the eye sockets (orbits), and the nose. The soft tissue in these areas, including the nerves, tendons, ligaments, salivary glands, blood vessels, and connective tissue, can also be injured.

Kids get so many bloody noses that we almost forget how serious they can be. The most frequently injured area of the face is the nose. It is also the most commonly missed fracture. A broken nose may not show up well on x-rays. A fracture of the nose may be associated with other injuries, such as a fracture around the eye or into the sinuses.

The second most common fracture of the face is the cheekbone (zygomatic arch). These usually are the result of a blow to the side of the face from an elbow or fist. Kids with this injury often have a flatness of the cheek area, and they can't open their mouths because the fracture fragments are preventing it.

A "blowout fracture" of the eye can occur after being hit in the face by a baseball or other object. The force of the blow is transmitted to the thin floor of the eye socket (orbit), resulting in the break or blowout. This often results in bleeding in or around the eye.

In general, if the player has a fracture, he or she will complain of severe pain at the site of the break. There will often be swelling and bruising of the soft tissue around the fracture, including black eyes. There may be a visible deformity if the fracture is complex and bone fragments separate enough to cause distortion of the face. The site will be very tender to the touch.

Bleeding from the nose or eyes often means there is some type of facial fracture. The player will be unable to bite normally. The face may become quite puffy.

Fractures of the lower jaw (mandible) are common facial fractures in sports. The TMJ (hinge joint of the jaw) is the joint that allows the jaw to open and close. The TMJ can be fractured or the joint can be disrupted by direct trauma such as a ball or stick hitting the face.

The player with a broken bone in the face needs to be checked for bleeding and swelling that could interfere with breathing. Ice packs can be applied to the face to decrease swelling and pain. The upper body should be lifted so the face is above the level of the heart. This can be done carefully with pillows or a blanket. This will reduce swelling and help prevent excess fluid from accumulating in the face.

But before the head is propped up, the player should be checked for a neck injury. Once the airway is checked and confirmed to be open, and it is confirmed that the player has not suffered any sort of nerve injury or concussion, the rest of the face can be examined for injury. This examination can be done by the team doctor or trainer. These players, once stabilized, are usually sent directly to the ER and then referred to a specialist.

As team doctors, my colleagues and I will check the skin of the face. We check for swelling, hematoma (accumulation of blood), and cuts. One of the most common sites for a cut is under the chin. This should alert the team doctor to the possibility of fractures of the lower jaw.

Another common site for a cut is to the side of the eye. The thin bone surrounding the eye (orbit) should be checked carefully for breaks. The face has a good supply of blood, so these lacerations usually bleed a lot, and pressure can be applied. The face is checked for areas of swelling, deformity, or tenderness. We want to look for any tears or lacerations in the mouth below the tongue, so the player will be asked to open his or her mouth. The examination should be done by the team doctor or trainer. The player will usually be taken to the ER and then follow up with a specialist.

Teeth should be examined for signs of broken teeth or abnormal bite. The doctor will have the player bite the teeth together. Any alteration of bite is abnormal. Three causes of an altered bite in injured players are a broken jaw, a jaw dislocation, or a tooth that is out of position. The examination can be done initially by the team doctor or trainer. The player should be sent to the ER and then follow up with the dentist.

Case Study: Meet SP, age sixteen; sport: soccer

"I was playing high school varsity soccer, defender, marking back, man to man when the injury occurred. I was running diagonal to the goal, toward the right about thirty yards out with another player on the right. When the goalie came out of the box, could not use his hands, the ball was bouncing, and I headed it away, but the goalie also tried to head the ball that I had already hit, and instead butted me right in the left side of my face.

"I immediately blacked out, and the next thing I remember is waking up, and the coach of the other team was over me, asking me if I was okay. I stood up and was light-headed and fell over. I was only alert for a few seconds, and I noticed that the lights were very bright (it was a night game). I had to squint. Everything was more intense and like I was in a tunnel.

"I felt stupid. I sat for a second on the sidelines, and I felt that the field and the coach seemed familiar. I was tough and wanted to play again. There was a volunteer doctor who suggested I sit on the sidelines. No examination was done, and I was given a ride home.

"When I got home, I got in the shower, blew my nose, and my whole face felt like it blew up with air. Fluid came out of my nose, and it was not snot. It was some other fluid. My face was like a balloon, and then the air came out of it. I thought there might be a problem. I called my family doctor, and he told me to go to sleep and see him in the morning. My aunt, who is an orthopedic surgeon, heard the story and called the doctor back and explained that she thought it was a facial fracture and concussion.

"My doctor then called back more urgent and told me to go to the ER. They did an immediate CT scan. The CT scan made me feel humble. The CT scan showed I had a mild concussion and orbital fracture.

It was recommended that I follow up with a plastic surgeon to make sure that it healed properly and straight. It took me about two weeks of feeling dumb and got *Ds* on my tests in school. I could not focus. The muscles in my face were messed up on the side of the face and could not smile properly for six months. I felt sleepy for a few weeks.

"I returned to sports two weeks later, before I was cleared. I was fine. Although, I was hesitant to do a header for a while. I feel fine now."

How to Prevent Dental and Facial Injuries

Players, coaches, and parents can take several steps to reduce the incidence of trauma to the face. Proper fitting headgear and face masks are important. Headgear is required in football, hockey, lacrosse, boxing, baseball, wrestling, and martial arts. All face masks and headgear should fit well. The face mask or shield should be fastened securely to the headgear, and the headgear should fit snugly on the player's head. The headgear should not flop around.

In the 1960s and 1970s mouth guards were used primarily in boxing and football. Today they are used in many more sports, including football, field hockey, ice hockey, wrestling, soccer, basketball, gymnastics, lacrosse, the martial arts, volleyball, boxing, and weightlifting. Mouth guards are close to 100 percent effective in preventing mouth injuries. Basketball, where mouth guards are not required, has a mouth injury rate of 34 percent. I rest my case.

Several types of mouth protectors are available:

- The stock mouth protector is intended to fit any mouth. They are available in a limited number of sizes and can be found in sporting goods stores and pharmacies. The stock mouth protector is the least expensive and does not need to be fitted by a doctor. The design of these protectors is the least desirable of all because they fit poorly. They can interfere with speech and breathing and require the mouth to remain closed in order for them to stay in place.

- The mouth-formed protector is commonly known as a "boil and bite." It is made of polyvinyl acetate. This mouth guard is preformed by the manufacturer in standard sizes. To make it fit a young athlete, at home you simply put it into boiling water for about one minute, then transfer to cold water for one second and immediately place it in the kid's mouth. As it cools, the plastic forms to the mouth and teeth.

- The advantages of this system are that it can be refitted if not properly fitted the first time (back into the boiling water), the cost is relatively low, and all fitting procedures can be accomplished at one sitting. The disadvantages include decreased retention (thinning from wear and tear) over time and hardening of the material from continued exposure to oral fluids. Studies have shown that because the occlusion (bite) is unbalanced when these are made, the stability of these guards is poor, and they cannot withstand the forces that can cause facial trauma.

- Custom mouth guards can be made by the dentist or a professional laboratory that the dentist gives instructions to. They accommodate children's mouths, braces, and bites that are changing because of growth. Some heavy contact sports such as football need a thicker guard. The custom-fitted guards fit more accurately, are more comfortable, and improve protection of the mouth. Most athletes playing contact sports will need a custom mouth guard. This option is my preferred choice. Cost is a factor. Sometimes these custom mouth guards can cost $500 to 2,000. But compare that to the cost of lost teeth or a broken jaw.

Regardless of the type of mouth guard used, many players think that mouth guards interfere with breathing. So you see kids spitting them out or taking them out. Like contact lens, they take some getting used to. Also, if there is not a good fit, or it is big and bulky, it will be hard to speak and breathe. Most dentists recommend wearing them only on the upper teeth.

A mouth guard, whether it is required in a sport or not, is an excellent investment in your kids' health. There is a much lower incidence of mouth injuries when mouth guards are used. Studies have shown that the incidence of fractured jaws and soft tissue injuries decreases significantly when mouth protection is used.

A study by Hickey and colleagues in 1967 used cadavers to show that when a blow to the chin was received, the mouth guard reduced the amplitude of the intracranial pressure wave and decreased the amount of bone deformation by 50 percent. This study shows that proper use of mouth guards can reduce the amount of trauma to the brain, decreasing the chance for concussion.

Finally, the psychological benefit of players knowing that there is a lower chance of their being hurt while wearing a mouth guard allows them to do what they are supposed to do, which is focus on playing. Coaches exert great influence on the players, and the players' behavior reflects the coach's opinion. This is especially true during practice. More injuries occur during practice than at any other time. It is imperative that coaches impress upon their athletes the need for mouth guard use at all times.

Many of the face and mouth injuries that occur in young athletes can significantly limit or end a young athlete's playing career. Quick and accurate on-site diagnosis and treatment is essential to minimizing potential damage from a face or mouth injury. The use of high-quality protective equipment is important if the players are going to perform at optimum levels in the safest manner possible. All organized sports teams, especially at the club and high school level, should have a team dentist available to them to promote oral health and safety.

BACKS, SPINES, AND PAIN IN KIDS

If you thought only Grandma had back pain, you would be incorrect. Kids experience injuries to their backs, but, unlike Grandma, their low back pain is rarely from anything specific and usually goes away without any treatment.

It is more likely that an athletic kid will have back problems than a kid who does not play sports. Athletes are simply doing more things that can expose a weakness in their bodies.

Pain in the lumbar spine (meaning lower part of the back) accounts for 5 to 8 percent of reported youth sports injuries. Although back pain is not the most common injury, it may be the most challenging to diagnose and treat.

Risks and Causes of Low Back Pain in Kids

- Excessive lifting and twisting leading to sprains and strains (most common cause)
- Growth spurts
- An abrupt increase in training intensity or frequency
- Poor technique
- Poorly fitting or broken sports equipment
- Leg-length inequality
- Poor core strength (Poor strength of the back and abdominal muscles and tightness in the lumbar spine or hamstrings and hip flexor muscles may contribute to low back pain.)
- Hits to the spine creating contusions or fractures (breaks) (Fractures in kids from severe injuries include compression fracture—from up and down loads—fracture of the growth plate, and lumbar vertebrae bone fractures/breaks.)

The large sacroiliac joint in the back part of the pelvis (upper buttock area) is also prone to irritation (it's also known as the SI joint). The signs and symptoms of a bulging disc (herniation) in youth may be less obvious than in adults. More unusual things like tumors and arthritis can occur, but this is rare in kids.

It is often difficult for kids to point to a specific spot for the back pain. The anatomy in this area is complex, and sometimes the nerves get irritated and move the pain around (this is called radiation pain). A thorough physical examination and description of what happened is helpful to make the diagnosis.

Doctors should order tests for the injured athlete who has long-term, severe problems, after a severe injury, or if there is no improvement with standard treatment. X-rays, bone scans, computed tomography (CT), and magnetic resonance imaging (MRI) can be used to help make the diagnosis.

What the Different Imaging Techniques Are

X-rays: X-rays use radiation to create a simple black-and-white image that looks like a film negative. It is useful for imaging bones, but not ligaments and tendons.

Bone scan: A bone scan is a nuclear scanning test that finds abnormalities in bones, such as fractures. This imaging can help diagnose fractures that are hard to see on an x-ray, such as a stress fracture. An injection, into a vein, of a small amount of radioactive material is required to obtain the image.

MRI: The MRI is the tunnel-like machine you often see on TV. This technique is used to show the internal structures of the body. MRI uses nuclear magnetic resonance to show the inside of the body. The patient lies in a large powerful magnet, and the magnetic field helps create the image by aligning the nuclei of the atoms in a certain way. We use it for imaging ligaments and tendons, for example.

CT: The CT or computed tomography scan (also called a CAT scan) is a medical image using radiation that employs computer-processed x-rays to produce the three-dimensional images or "slices." This test gives us excellent visuals of the bones of the body. However, the exposure to radiation with a CT scan is about ten to a hundred times more than a chest x-ray.

Most low back pain in a kid responds to standard treatment. Prompt treatment of a new injury should include ice, electrical stimulation, anti-inflammatory medications (such as ibuprofen), and gentle exercises. Let's take each one:

- Apply ice. Ice can be used for therapy to reduce pain and inflammation. Usually it is not used for more than ten to fifteen minutes at a time on the injured limb. It is very useful when an injury first occurs (in the first seventy-two hours). A bag of frozen peas is a wonderful ice bag. It can mold to the low back (and very well for a shin or shoulder or elbow, for that matter). Wrap it in a dish towel to keep ice from direct contact with skin.

- Electrical stimulation uses electrical currents to decrease pain and promote healing. This is delivered by a machine and usually by a physical therapist. It can also be used to strengthen a muscle and promote blood flow for healing.

- Ask your doctor about dosing for anti-inflammatory medications. Nonsteroidal anti-inflammatory drugs (NSAIDs) such as ibuprofen are a class of medication that can help with pain relief and decrease swelling. Many of these are available in any drugstore over the counter. The instructions on the bottle should be followed. Report any side effects to a doctor.

- Gentle exercises to reduce low back pain are not complicated and can usually be done at home or with a physical therapist. Too little activity can lead to loss of flexibility, strength, and endurance. Do not let your injured athlete miss school and simply lie in bed. Easy exercises include hamstring stretching, yoga, and Pilates. Back and abdominal muscles should be strengthened to help the body maintain an upright position and movement. Abdominal exercises can be done with an exercise ball, which is portable. Ask a trainer or physical therapist to show how to do easy exercises at home.

- Bed rest is not advised because the player can get weak very quickly. An early strengthening program can include core strengthening, flexion exercises, extension exercises, and Pilates. None of this activity should cause pain.

An injured athlete should not return to practice until he or she can do it without pain. The player should have a full or almost full range of motion without pain and have regained enough strength in the muscles related to the sport. Endurance needs to also be regained.

After a sprain or strain this period of time may only be a few days. For a stress fracture of the lower back, however, the return to sports may take around six months. Be patient because the risk of reinjury is great.

During this period of time gentle exercises and low-impact exercises such as cycling should be done. When the athlete does return, inform the coach of any limitations. Your doctor is your guide here.

The return to practice and play may take place in stages. An injured kid might go back to practices and drills, but not to the rougher parts of the sport. Injured athletes need to be encouraged to take more breaks, stretch, warm up, and keep at low intensity for the first few weeks back. Kids need to listen to their bodies (not to their eagerness to play).

If they have pain, that's a danger sign. A little soreness after a workout is expected. Direct any questions to the doctor and ask what you, as a parent or coach, should do next for the injured player.

A study of 2,846 patients noted that 75 percent of the kids with low back pain had a mechanical origin for the problem, such as poor strength in core muscles and pelvis. The average age of athletes in this study was around fourteen, and 63 percent of them were girls. If there was a diagnosis, it was commonly (in 7 percent of kids) spondylolysis (where part of the bone of the lower spine weakens and breaks) (Miller 2011).

Back Conditions Explained

Both spondylolisthesis (a slip in the bone) and spondylolysis (a break in the bone) can cause back pain in the young athlete. Don't worry if the doctor uses these big words. Here's what they mean:

Spondylolysis: Spondylolysis often results from an injury or from repetitive bending, twisting, or loading of the back muscles and bones. It is thought to be a stress fracture (break) in part of the vertebrae bone called the pars interarticularis. This can cause low back pain. Spondylolysis is commonly seen in kids who play soccer, football, weight lifting, gymnastics, wrestling, volleyball, diving, and basketball.

Spondylolisthesis: The condition involves defects of a vertebra's *pars interarticularis* (spondylolysis) and the slippage of one vertebra in relation to another vertebra. Spondylolisthesis is often associated with syndyloysis.

Spondylolysis is a defect in part of the lumbar vertebrae (back bones) in the spine. It is thought to be a stress fracture (break) in part of the vertebrae bone called the pars interarticularis. Spondylolysis often results from a back injury or from repetitive bending, twisting, or loading of the back muscles and bones. This can cause low back pain. Spondylolysis is commonly seen in kids who play soccer, football, weight lifting, gymnastics, wrestling, volleyball, diving and basketball.

This condition is often thought to be a sprain or strain at first. For this reason, the condition can sometimes be ignored or missed for a period of time. X-rays are often normal, which is why advanced imaging studies such as bone scans, MRI, and a CT scan may be necessary to make the diagnosis.

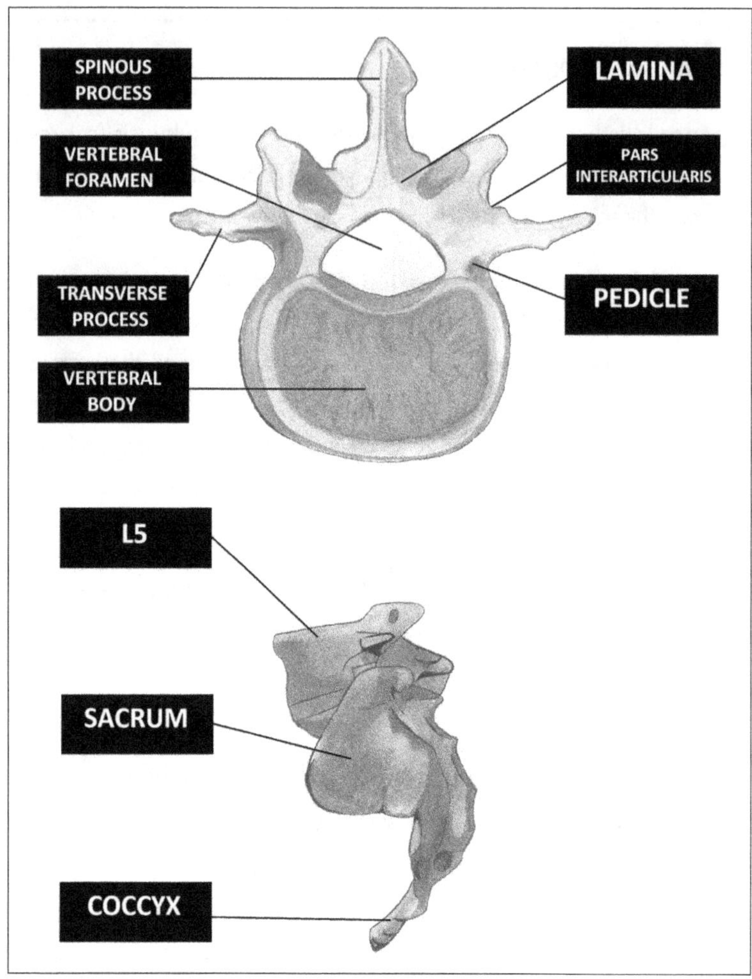

Anatomy of the Vertebrae.

This type of back injury is more common during growth spurts when there is more stress on the bone. The stress fracture that results may be a complete or incomplete fracture (for clarification, a complete fracture breaks all the way through the bone, and the incomplete fracture does not).

In about 15 percent of *pars interarticularis* stress injuries, and resultant fractures, there is a progression to spondylolisthesis (a forward slipping of the vertebrae on each other).

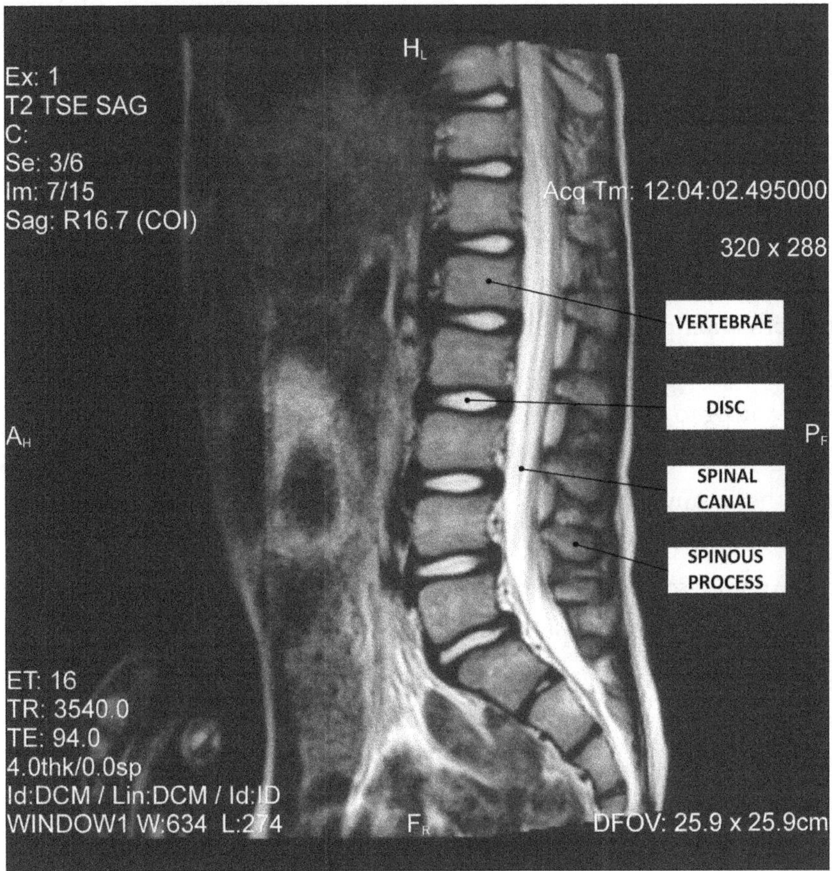

Anatomy of the lumbar spine. The MRI shows vertebral bodies, discs, spinal processes, and spinal canal.

Recovery requires a period of relative rest, ice, medication, and strength and conditioning exercises. It is important the young athlete work on flexibility and strength. Strengthening of the trunk (core) muscles is a very important part of rehabilitation.

The repeated stress of running, jumping, and bending activity can then produce a stress (also known as a fatigue) fracture. The athlete needs to rest or the fracture will get worse and result in a complete fracture. This can then lead to a persistent problem. Sometimes the bone does not heal (this is called a nonunion). Activity must be restricted until the bone is healed.

In some cases, a brace may be helpful to rest the back and control pain. In mild cases, the problem can be treated like a sprain or strain. In severe cases it may take about six months to return to sports. It is rare for surgery to be required.

If there is a slip in the vertebrae (spondylolisthesis), there are special things to think about. A player who has less than a 50 percent forward slip can usually return to all sports when he or she is pain free and after a good rehabilitation program. If there is a forward slip of 50 percent or greater, it may be recommended that the athlete change sports to something less aggravating to the injury.

Players with a spondylolisthesis (slipping) should be checked every six months for any more forward slipping. This is especially important to get periodic checks during growth spurts.

Another somewhat common problem seen in the young athlete with back pain is juvenile kyphosis. This pain may seem to be in the middle of the back (not the low back), and it most likely occurs during puberty. (This is different from curvature of the spine or scoliosis, the "S" spine.) Kyphosis may be from a stress fracture of the vertebrae, osteoporosis, hereditary causes, or birth defects.

The athlete, in this case, will have a round back deformity that gets worse with forward bending. A diagnosis is made by x-ray. The vertebrae will look like wedges that are compressed in the front as the back bends forward.

The goal of treatment in most cases is to relieve the symptoms. Treatment should make the player feel better. Extension exercises for the back and good posture are recommended. A brace may help the player with symptoms. The back "bump," however, will not go away with this treatment. Sometimes surgery is necessary if the deformity is big and the pain won't go away.

As with all back injuries, a complete rehabilitation program is very important prior to the athlete returning to sports.

A disc injury is a relatively uncommon cause of back pain in young players. Back pain from a disc injury may or may not be associated with sciatica (pain that shoots down the leg). A good physical examination and history of the injury will help the doctor make the diagnosis. An MRI can also be helpful to diagnose a disc problem in kids.

The treatment of a disc injury in kids is similar to the treatment in adults. Epidural injections are usually not necessary for the young athlete. But surgery may be recommended if symptoms continue after a complete rehabilitation program. The good news, however, is that surgery is not usually necessary in young athletes with a disc injury.

BACK INJURIES: NOT GLAMOROUS BECAUSE YOU DON'T EVEN GET A CAST

Although not common, low back injuries do occur in young athletes. I had one athlete tell me that he would rather have an injury that required a cast because at least you "looked" injured.

Sprains of the back ligaments and strains of the muscles of the back are the most common back injuries in the young athlete. More serious injuries that occur in athletic kids may feel like a sprain. Repetitive overuse, flexion, and rotation, discussed later in this chapter, can cause problems in the young spine.

In summary, a thorough examination and medical history that includes how the injury may have happened can help us doctors make the proper diagnosis. Imaging studies such as x-rays, MRI, CT scans, and bone scans are sometimes necessary.

A kid with a significant back injury may feel fine at rest and worse with activity. The pain may come and go. But if the pain does not go away after two weeks of standard treatment such as ice, pain medication, rehabilitation, and rest, the child should see a specialist and obtain an x-ray or other imaging and further testing if necessary.

Specialists might be an orthopedic spine surgeon or a neurosurgeon. Both specialize in this area. If there is a neurological disorder or weakness, the child is more likely to work with a neurosurgeon. Your family doctor can refer you.

Once the pain is controlled, the young athlete should be shown, by the doctor or a physical therapist, a proper strength and conditioning program for recovery and to prevent future problems. Flexibility and strength are emphasized, especially for the back and the core muscles. Exercises are also given for sport-specific muscles to improve performance. I discuss these types of rehab later in this book.

Patients don't want to hear this, but a significant back injury may require a one- to three-month rest period from sports to heal.

Athletes who take time off from a sport must also remember to stay fit. They should perform low-intensity cardiovascular exercises, such as riding a stationary bike at least three times a week for thirty minutes. Otherwise, there will be a decrease in stamina. This, in turn, will make it difficult to return to sports and put the player at risk for another injury.

Proper rehabilitation will also help the player not be discouraged during the initial return to play. Before the student athlete is released to play, sport-specific exercises are important. Sport-specific exercises mirror the activities of the specific sport. This should include warm-ups, cool down, quick footwork, balance, coordination, and core strengthening.

Pilates is an excellent activity for many of my young patients with back problems. No exercise should cause pain. And all exercise should be monitored by a trained medical specialist (a spine surgeon or a physical therapist). Poor technique, mechanics, and habits need to be corrected. Aerobic conditioning needs to be maintained throughout treatment for back injuries under the supervision of the doctor.

A young athlete's body is constantly changing because of growth and maturation. The injured young athlete will, therefore, be different on an anatomic and physiologic level when he or she returns to play. This should work to the player's advantage.

Why is that? Kids get bigger and stronger. The bigger and stronger muscle mass will protect the injured part. The more mature player will now be able to recognize when there is something wrong and stop playing and seek treatment. The neuromuscular reaction time increases as the body matures as well. Or so we hope!

Case Study: Meet JJ, age fifteen; sport: basketball

"It all started three or four years ago when I was playing at the Anaheim Sports Center. Some of the guys weren't there; as a result, I and several other of my teammates got some more playing time. We were down with a couple seconds to go, and I went in for a little five-footer to tie it up. Not only did I miss the shot, but my lower back started hurting really bad. It stayed like that for about three weeks before going away.

"I could tell my teammates didn't believe me, and as a result, I was looked down upon. It wasn't too bad, but it never feels good to be limited physically, no matter how long the injury lasts. After that, the pain was off and on for a year or two, but then it came back in a big way. I could play through it, but the pain was severe, and it was holding me back. "

JJ has had three MRIs and CT scans, which showed a stress fracture of the lumbar spine (spondylolysis). Over time the images showed progressive healing. He started doing Pilates twice a week and low-impact cardiovascular training on a stationary bike. He used a bone stimulator, a device that is used to promote bone healing with low-dose electrical current or ultrasound, and increased his intake of vitamin D and calcium. He did not play basketball for three months and was lucky that the injury occurred early in the season his sophomore year. He had time to heal, rehabilitate, and get back in the game.

JJ missed most of his sophomore year and felt that, because of good teamwork, practice, good character, strength, and conditioning, he was advanced to the varsity level by the end of the year. He was named captain for being a leader on the team, not just a great basketball player. And he was voted most inspirational player on the team by his fellow players and coaches (and there's a lesson in that alone).

Case Study: Meet TR, age sixteen; sport: basketball

It all started during JV basketball practice one night. TR was playing in a scrimmage, and out of nowhere, he felt a sharp pain in his lower back. At first he thought that it was a spasm of some sort and would be a sometime deal. However, after feeling this pain several more times in the following weeks, he started getting worried.

He felt that his JV coaches believed that he was injured, and noted that they allowed him to go see the trainer whenever it was necessary. He also said that the spasms were becoming less frequent after his season ended. TR treated himself with Advil and ice. He was diagnosed with a low back sprain. He had no treatment other than stretching and ice.

Case Study: Meet GO, age sixteen; sport: basketball

GO thinks the problem started in eighth grade after lifting some heavy weights. GO said that he felt a sharp pain in his lower back, specifically on the right side. He immediately thought that it wasn't a serious issue, but after feeling the pain in his back for weeks on end, he began to realize that it might be a long-term injury. He noticed that others were criticizing his lack of toughness and commenting on the fact that young people don't get injuries.

It has gone away to a certain extent, but he will still feel it while doing heavy squats. GO believes that the pain will subside once he is done growing. His symptoms are consistent with a stress fracture of the lumbar spine (spondylolysis) and an MRI is recommended.

Case Study: Meet JP, age seventeen; sport: sailing

JP was sixteen when the back pain started when he was sailing as a member of the crew, hiking out, and he had a sharp pain in his lower back. The pain went away in three weeks. Four months later, while playing high school varsity soccer, and after a summer of extreme growth, JP felt pain in his back during play. He was playing in the position of outside fullback. JP made no change in the intensity of his play, but when he ran he had soreness on his right side.

"I thought something was wrong with my hip at first and that I could play through the pain. I thought I would outgrow the pain. I took time off and got out of shape and made it worse. The back pain was not getting better, even with rest, and eventually I got an MRI. The MRI showed a stress fracture, and a slip of the back bones" (spondylolisthesis and spondylolysis with slight impingement on the spinal cord).

"PT was prescribed and core strengthening, and it took a long time, but I got through the growth spurt. I started running after growth stopped, but it would hurt after I ran. Then I went to a spine specialist who recommended a surgery called a flexible fusion. After that surgery I actually felt worse for about one and a half years. Then I concentrated on yoga and core strengthening, and the pain went away. I can now run without pain and have returned to club soccer."

These stories are all from high school–level male players who suffered a stress fracture of the lumbar spine. Their stories are similar: they thought the problem would just go away or that it was just a back strain.

SHOULDERS AND ELBOWS

We're moving down the body to shoulders and elbows. And this is where things get complicated.

Muscles, ligaments, joint capsule, labrum, and tendons all surround the shoulder. Working in concert, they all contribute to function, motion, and stability. Think fastball pitcher (because of throwing) or spiking the volleyball (hitting overhead). And because of all these movements in all directions, the shoulder can be injured in many different ways. In fact, all the structures I just mentioned can be injured.

Here's a little anatomy lesson: the shoulder joint, also called the glenohumeral joint, is complicated. The humeral head (ball) sits in the socket called the glenoid fossa. The glenoid fossa is a shallow socket, and an extra ring of tissue called the glenoid labrum is attached to the edge to make it more deep and stable. In addition, the shoulder joint is also surrounded by a capsule, which connects bone to bone and makes the joint more stable. The shoulder moves in all directions.

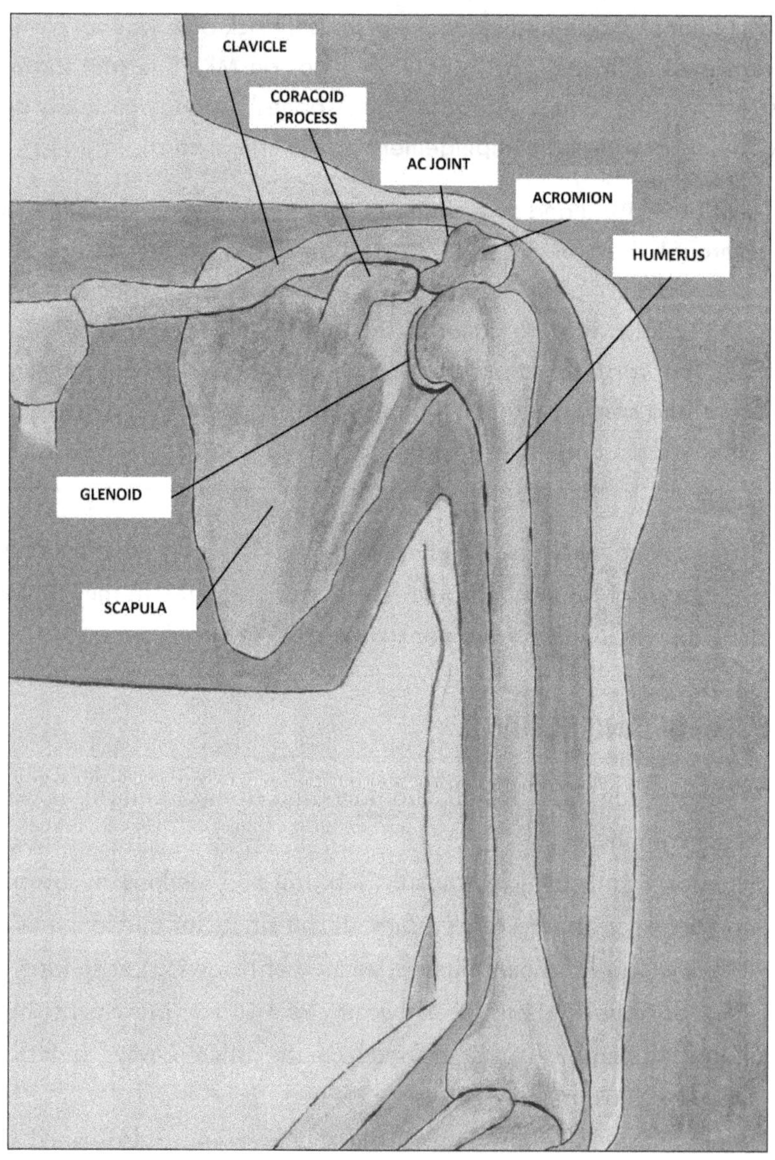

Anatomy of the Shoulder, from the Front.

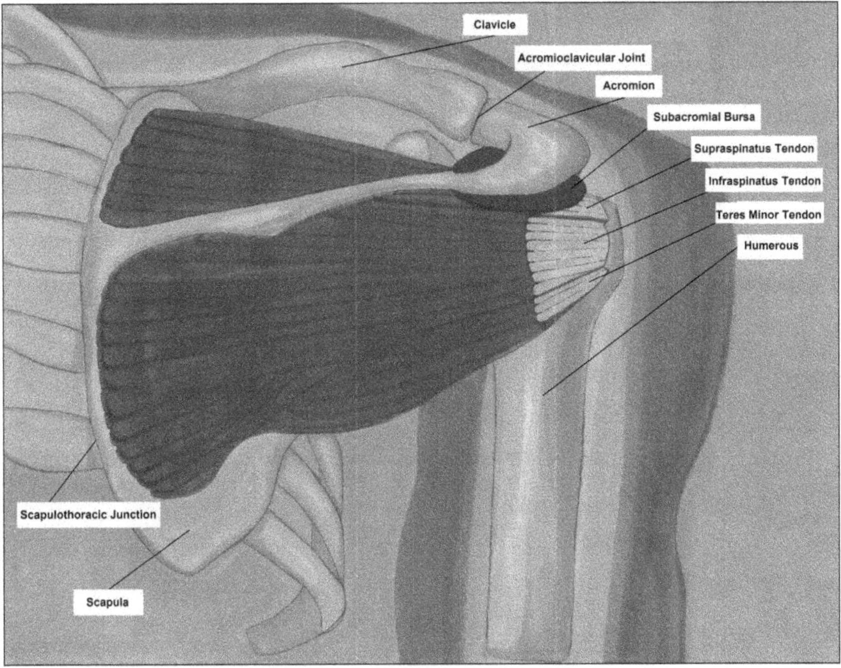

Anatomy of the Shoulder, from the Back.

I mention these medical terms because you may find yourself sitting in an exam room or ER (let's hope not), and a doctor may use the technical medical terms. You have two options: You can know the anatomy ahead of time, which most people don't. Or you (as the parent or athlete) can stop the doctor, and it's perfectly acceptable to say, "I'm not familiar with these medical terms. Can you explain my injury in simpler terms? Can you draw me a picture? Would you point this out on my x-ray?"

If you're going to recover from any injury, or help your child get back in the game, it's important to know what you're dealing with. See it, feel it, and know the goal in rehab.

Common Shoulder Injuries

The rotator cuff, shoulder joint capsule, ligaments, and the biceps tendon help stabilize the shoulder. The stabilization from the structures, other than bone, is important because the shoulder joint has a shallow socket.

(In our quick course of anatomy, a tendon is a tough band of connective tissue that connects muscle to bone. Ligaments connect a bone to other bones. Both can be injured.)

If a young athlete has problems with moving the shoulder away from the body, called abduction and external rotation, this can be a sign of a condition called anterior instability, which is the most common type of shoulder instability. Anterior instability of the shoulder can be a result of an injury (such as a shoulder dislocation) or repetitive motion and possibly poor mechanics or technique.

Some kids just have loose joints and even dislocate their shoulders at will (Hertling and Kessler 1996). Sometimes surgery is necessary to repair the injured tissue and correct the instability.

Athletes with anterior instability of the shoulder should not overstretch the structures at the front (anterior) of the shoulder. Shoulder abduction and external rotation (away from the body similar to throwing a baseball) should not be forced. This has been called the "high-five" position and should be avoided during training (Fees et al. 1998).

Athletes with this type of injury will want to modify their strength training on machines, and I offer some tips in the chapter on strength and conditioning.

Instability of the back (posterior) part of the shoulder is less common than anterior instability. Injury may occur when the shoulder is flexed forward, and the arm is rotated internally (thumbs down). For example, in football, when an offensive lineman blocks another player, the lineman's arm can be in a position of about 90 degrees forward flexion, and his elbow is completely straight (extended). The ball (humeral head) of his shoulder joint is pushed to the back (posterior) of the socket (glenoid) as he completes the movement of pushing (Wilk, Andrews, and Arrigo 1997). This position puts a lot of stress on the back (posterior) shoulder socket and joint.

Strengthening the rotator cuff and scapular muscles may be the most important thing that the young athlete does to prevent injury (see chapter on strength and conditioning).

Case Study: Chris, fourteen years old, sport: volleyball

Chris was an up-and-coming club volleyball player who also was on the high school freshman team. A tall kid, he was six feet four at just fourteen. Chris was a powerful outside hitter with some serious hops. He was playing volleyball about two to three hours a day when he noticed that it hurt even to lift his arm after practice, and it felt heavy. He did not have pain during play, at first, and he did not recall a specific injury. He was a super aggressive hitter and was told he had "more rotation than normal" in his shoulder. He thought that was a good thing. He was such a force on the team that the coach did not rotate him out very much. Needless to say, he went right out of the high school season and into club without a break, and the pain got worse.

He thought if he rested for a few days, the shoulder would get better, so he sat out for ten days and then played in a beach tournament. The second day of the tournament, the shoulder started to hurt during play. The pain was mainly in the front and on the side of the shoulder.

His mom was in the medical field and got him in to see a physical therapist who used ice, ultrasound, electrical stimulation, and the same strengthening program that all baseball pitchers do. The shoulder got better at first, but when he returned to practice with his trainer, the pain returned.

Chris finally went to see a shoulder specialist, who recommended that he get an MRI. The MRI was to check out if there was a tear of the rotator cuff or cartilage (labrum) around the shoulder. He was told that if the MRI showed a tear, then surgery was necessary, as his rehab with the physical therapist had not helped. Unfortunately, there was a tear of the labrum, and surgery was recommended. After the surgery he was told that he would not be able to play volleyball for three to twelve months. Chris, his parents and his coach were disappointed but knew that it could happen.

He went back to physical therapy after the surgery to decrease pain and swelling and improve the strength of the muscles around the shoulder, just like baseball pitchers do. Sadly, Chris had a long recuperation period and had to sit out the rest of the next high school season as the shoulder repaired itself. Even though he sat on the bench at every game during the season while he was recovering, Chris was an inspiration to his teammates.

At first, he returned to play in the back row, not raising his arms above shoulder level. Eventually he fully recovered. He presently is a starter on a nationally ranked club and high school varsity team. He has returned to the outside hitter position.

The lesson is this: Most players return to their sport. And sometimes it takes a while to get back in the game. But when a properly rehabbed athlete does return, he or she should come back a more mature player—physically and mentally.

As I mentioned, any and all of the structures that comprise the complicated shoulder can be injured. Now to the shoulder ligaments. The glenoid labrum (the fibrocartilage-gristle-like ring attached to the rim of the shoulder socket (glenoid) to deepen the shoulder joint) is the main spot for the shoulder ligaments to attach. A SLAP (superior labrum antero-posterior) lesion may occur during a fall onto an outstretched hand or shoulder.

A SLAP can result in a tear or inflammation of the rotator cuff. SLAP injuries can occur after a baseball player slides or falls down during a fielding play. The injured player will commonly complain of pain during motion that requires the shoulder to be placed in abduction (away from the body), external rotation (thumbs up) or extension (high-five position).

The two most common traumatic injuries around the elbow are fracture or dislocation. The mechanism of injury is commonly direct trauma (a blow or hit) or falling on an outstretched straight (extended) arm. We initially treat the fracture or the dislocation on the field by splinting the arm in the position in which it is found. No attempts should be made to correct the deformity except by the medical doctor.

Let's move down the arm to the wrists and fingers where sports injuries are quite common.

WRISTS AND HANDS (AND FINGERS)

The vast majority of wrist and hand injuries are traumatic, and most are fractures (breaks). Fractures involve the radius and the ulna (the two bones in the forearm), the scaphoid (small bone in the wrist), the metacarpals (hand bones), and the phalanges (fingers).

Injuries almost always happen by direct trauma—hitting a wall with a hand or closed fist or landing on an outstretched hand, even jamming a finger against the ball, for example. Deformity may not be obvious, but swelling and tenderness are almost always the first signs of a fracture.

The initial treatment is splinting and ice. X-rays are required. Setting the broken bone in the right position (this process is called reduction) and immobilization in a splint or cast are the most common treatments. Surgery is much less likely in a child or adolescent athlete than in an adult. The player may return to the sport after healing and rehabilitation, and the time it takes to rehab depends on the exact injury and how serious it is.

Finger and thumb dislocations are common. They may be accompanied by a fracture. Dislocations should be splinted and only reduced (put back in place) by a medical doctor. If a finger seems out of joint, splint it on the field and see a doctor. This is one of those do-not-try-this-at-home procedures, please.

X-rays are mandatory to see what's going on (in case there is a fracture along with the dislocation). The doctor will usually splint the injury for seven to ten days. Of course, if the bone is broken too, the splinting time will be longer. Breaks take longer to heal than dislocations.

Most fractures and dislocations can be treated with manipulation (setting the fracture) and immobilization. Occasionally, surgery with or without fixation (screws, pins, and plates) is necessary to treat these injuries and straighten out the bone.

The most common ligament injury is to the ulnar collateral ligament of the thumb. These are the ligaments that hold bone to bone on the sides of the thumb joints. There can be a ligament injury as well as a growth plate fracture. Physical examination and x-rays are required, and a stress x-ray may be necessary for diagnosis. A cast or a splint for a minimum of four to six weeks is necessary. Surgery is not common.

Jersey finger is the most common tendon injury of the hand and wrist in the young athlete. This occurs when a player gets his fingers stuck in another player's jersey. The player and coach usually assume that there is a sprain. The injury is a partial or complete rupture of the flexor tendon to the finger. The big clue about this injury is that the player is unable to make a fist normally. This injury can only be corrected with surgery. If this injury is not corrected, it can be difficult or impossible to correct later.

That's the upper half of the body. Now let's move down to the lower half.

LEG INJURIES

We know our kids are growing by leaps and bounds when we try to stay ahead of keeping them in shoes that fit their ever-growing feet, like puppies developing into their monster-sized paws. And we wonder if their pants shrank in the wash.

Injuries to the legs and feet of growing athletes—as with other parts of the immature body—are often unique to kids. A large range of injuries can occur in the immature young athlete that involve the growth plate, growing bones, and soft tissues that are quickly changing.

Growth plates in kids get put under extra stress during sports. Because these areas are also growing, and the bones are getting longer, kids may be less flexible. In other words, kids may be at risk for injury just because the bones are getting longer and putting more stretch on the soft tissues, among other reasons.

Muscle injuries such as strains and contusions (hits and blows) are common in adolescents and young athletes. Muscle strains are commonly associated with poor (or no) warm-ups, overuse, fatigue, history of previous injury, climate, and surface conditions. The thigh muscles are a common area of injury for strains as well. A strain is a muscle pull or even a muscle tear, which implies damage to the muscle.

Injury to the bones of the legs usually occurs at the weakest link—the epiphyseal plate (the growth plate). A well-known classification system for determining the significance of these injuries is called the Salter-Harris classification. The higher the number, the more serious the fracture.

- The type 1 and 2 fractures have a good outcome if in a good position (reduced) and protected until healed (with a cast, for example).
- The type 3 and 4 (the bones are more displaced, moved) can require surgery to place in the right (anatomic) position. The type 3 and 4 are carefully followed throughout growth to make sure the growth plate does not close (stop growing) early or in an irregular way.

The knee is the largest and most complicated joint in the body. The knee is made of bones called the femur (thighbone), tibia (shinbone) and the patella (kneecap).

The knee is stabilized by four major ligaments (remember, these attach bone to bone):

- Medial collateral ligament (on the inside) or MCL
- Lateral collateral ligament (on the outside) or LCL
- Two cruciate ligaments (the crossed ligaments in the center of the knee), referred to as the anterior cruciate ligament (ACL) and the posterior cruciate ligament (PCL)

The articular cartilage is the slippery surface of the joint where the femur and the tibia come together. Cartilage is much slicker than ice on ice and allows the knee to glide smoothly through its range of motion. The meniscus, made up of another type of cartilage, is actually a firm but rubbery disc between the two bones that make up the knee joint. There is both a medial (inside) and a lateral (outside) meniscus in each knee. The meniscus is a shock absorber for the knee.

Everyone has known someone who has had surgery to correct a problem knee, so the terms *ACL* and *meniscus* may be somewhat familiar. Or Grandma got a new knee because she was walking with such pain, "bone on bone."

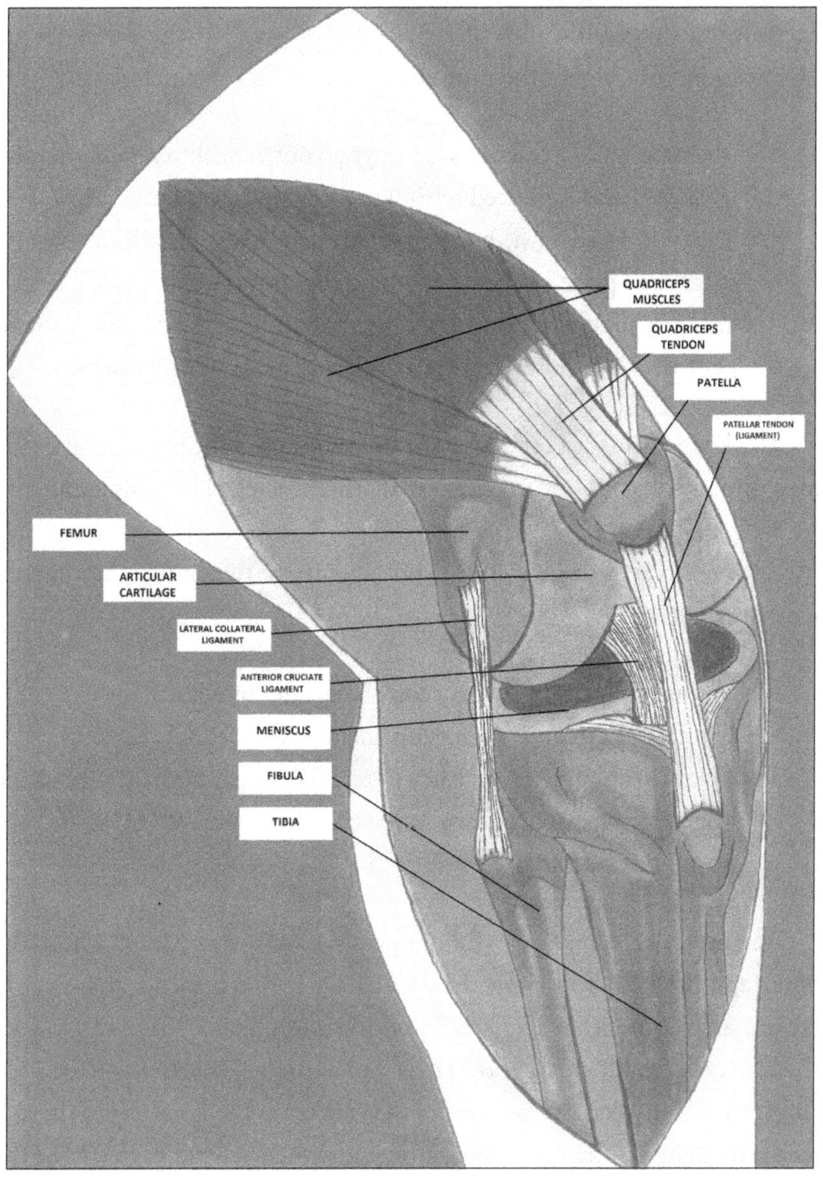

Anatomy of the Knee.

Although knee problems in adulthood come with the grace of aging, the incidence of knee injuries in all children and adolescents has increased significantly in recent years (Sampson et al. 2001). In kids, anterior cruciate and meniscal tears have grown in the period from 1999 to 2010, with a 400 percent increase in ACL tears. Much of the increase has been in the last five years. Other knee injuries are on the rise also.

A study from Children's Hospital of Philadelphia (*Science Daily*) has reported an increase in children requiring knee surgery. Even before the studies started showing this trend, we doctors saw it coming. The increase in knee injuries and surgery goes along with the increase in intensity and participation by kids in sports. Also, kids are specializing sooner and playing year-round in their sport. That did not happen twenty years ago.

At the same time, kids are playing as if they are professionals, with more intensity, over a longer season. Again, this wasn't the case twenty years ago.

However, it should be pointed out that there has also been an improvement in diagnostic testing over time. It is also more common for aggressive treatment of these injuries in kids.

The treatment for a broken bone (a fracture) is a splint in the position in which the limb is found if the injury occurs during sport action. If there is a significant deformity present—and you will know when the knee looks out of place, for example—only a medical doctor should reduce (correct) the deformity. Ice should be applied immediately on the field or court where the child is injured.

Expect the medical evaluation to include x-rays. Sometimes a stress x-ray or MRI and CT scan are necessary to make an accurate diagnosis and treatment plan.

Fractures about the knee can be quite serious, and if there is serious deformity, arteries, veins, and nerves around the knee can be damaged. Although most fractures can be straightened and then put into a cast, sometimes surgery is necessary to align the bone. Sometimes screws, plates, and pins need to be used to hold the bone straight. This is called internal fixation.

The athlete is allowed to return to play only when the fracture has completely healed. Rehabilitation with physical therapy and a sport-specific program (drills and skills associated with the sport) are usually necessary before the kid returns to sports.

The meniscus is a shock absorber of the knee. The most common mechanism of injury to this structure is a twisting injury with a fixed foot and hyperflexion (bending) of the knee. It can bring tears to your eyes just thinking about a child's leg getting twisted.

The athlete will complain of delayed and recurrent swelling, pain at the joint line of the knee, and catching and locking (which simply means the knee gets stuck in a position and has to be manipulated to get out of it; there is not a smooth back and forth motion of the knee).

The diagnosis of a meniscus tear is made based on history and physical examination. X-rays do not show the meniscus but should be taken to make sure that there is no injury to the bone. MRI is often used to make the diagnosis.

Many medical studies show that when a portion of the meniscus is removed, the articular cartilage (smooth surface of the bones where they come together to make the joint) that the meniscus protects will wear down faster than normal. This will result in the early onset of arthritis or degenerative joint disease. Therefore, everything possible should be done to keep the meniscus.

A meniscus tear generally requires surgery, but unless there is locking and recurrent catching, nonoperative care is an option. The nonoperative care is PRICE MM (see the boxed explanation) and rehabilitation.

You will be referred to the PRICE MM care often as we move through other types of injuries.

PRICE MM

PRICE MM is an acronym that stands for Protect, Rest, Ice, Compression, Elevation, and two more aspects called Modalities and Medication. This is the type of home care that can help certain injuries either when they happen or after a doctor has sent the patient home after treatment.

Post these instructions where you keep your medicines or program them into your smartphone so if someone gets injured at a game or elsewhere, you'll know what to do. As always, seek emergency medical care if you're in doubt about what's going on with an injury.

Protect: Protect the area of the injury with a cast, brace, or sling as necessary.

Rest: Limit the use of the injured area. Severe injuries may require complete rest, but less severe may allow rehabilitation and cross-training.

Ice: Ice is applied to the injured area for twenty minutes or less to decrease inflammation. This may be done during the first seventy-two hours of an acute injury. Ice is usually recommended about three or more times a day, but don't overdo the time that the ice is applied to the limb. Ice should not be applied directly onto the skin, or you can risk frostbite.

Compression: Compression will help limit the amount of inflammation to the injured area. Compression is used to reduce the swelling that results from injury and inflammation. An elastic bandage (ACE bandage) is commonly used. The fit should be snug so the limb doesn't move freely yet allows blood flow.

Elevation: Elevation helps increase blood return to the heart. This will help decrease swelling. So if the injury is a foot, lie on the couch and prop the foot up on the arm of the couch with pillows. An injured arm can be elevated on top of several pillows for someone lying down.

Modalities: Ice, heat, ultrasound, phonophoresis, and iontophoresis. These techniques are usually applied by a physical therapist or athletic trainer and help decrease swelling and pain, and speed recovery. (Iontophoresis is electromotive drug administration through a technique that uses small electric charges to deliver a medicine through the skin. It can be thought of as an injection without needles. It is used for decreasing inflammation. Phonophoresis uses ultrasound to deliver topical medication and to enhance the absorption of the topical medication. This is used to decrease pain and swelling.)

Medicine: Nonsteroidal anti-inflammatories (NSAID) medications can be used to help limit swelling and pain. They can be purchased over the counter or with a prescription. Examples of NSAIDs are ibuprofen (the generic name). Tylenol (acetaminophen) is not an NSAID.

In general, if the athlete becomes pain free on this PRICE MM program, a trial return to sports may be begun with the doctor's release. If the symptoms return, surgery may be considered. The surgery is done with an arthroscope (a small fiber-optic camera placed into the knee) through small incisions. Every effort is made to repair (sew back together) the meniscus. The majority of tears can be repaired, but sometimes they have to be trimmed back to where they are torn.

Rehabilitation should follow this surgery. A full range of motion, strength equal to the noninjured side, and the ability to perform sport-specific activity is required for the player to return to the field.

The articular cartilage—that slippery surface that allows a smooth motion of the knee joint—can become injured in the same way the meniscus is injured. Isolated injury to the articular cartilage is less likely than injury to the meniscus.

Articular cartilage injuries are difficult to diagnose. The athlete will complain of pain, swelling, and locking and catching just like the meniscus injury. X-rays will not show articular cartilage damage unless bone is also injured. So an MRI is usually necessary to make the diagnosis. With an MRI, we can actually see the ligaments, the tendons, the cartilage, and the meniscus.

Occasionally, there can be an injury involving both articular cartilage and the bone to which the cartilage is attached. This injury is called osteochondritis dessicans (OCD).

Injury to articular cartilage that has catching or locking of the knee will usually require surgery, which can be done with the arthroscope. The injured area is usually trimmed out so that it does not catch or lock.

Suspected OCD must be evaluated with an MRI or CT scan. If the injured area is not detached, it usually can be treated without surgery but will require crutches and a period of time where the athlete cannot put weight on the leg. Rehabilitation is usually recommended.

If the injured cartilage is partially attached, or especially if fully detached, surgery is usually necessary for possible reattachment of the piece. Articular cartilage injuries cannot be ignored, especially if OCD is present. These injuries can be difficult to treat, even in the best hands. Be aware that surgery is not always successful, and the athlete may be unable to return to sports activity.

Ligament Injuries: Save the ACL

Let's talk about ligament injuries. Ligaments attach bone to bone and provide stability to a joint. An injury to the ligament is called a sprain. There are three grades of injury to a ligament.

- Grade I sprain is an injury to the substance of the ligament causing pain but minimal or no instability. (Instability means laxity or increased motion, which is not normal. The knee joint may feel as if it is giving out, if it is unstable, for example.)
- Grade II sprain is a stretch injury to the ligament with a partial tear causing moderate instability.
- Grade III sprain is a complete tear of the ligament and is associated with significant instability.

The medial collateral ligament of the knee (MCL) is the most common injury to a ligament around the knee. The medial collateral ligament and the lateral collateral ligament are most often injured by direct trauma such as an impact from the side (think football tackle here). The athlete will complain of swelling, pain, and instability on the inside (MCL) or outside of the knee (LCL).

Immediate treatment is PRICE MM, crutches, and splinting. X-rays are required to rule out a fracture. Ongoing treatment is PRICE MM and a functional hinge-brace. A hinged knee brace provides increased support and stability to the knee—more than an elastic brace or neoprene sleeve. The hinged brace is dynamic and allows movement so the knee does not get stiff.

An injured kid may return to play when there is no pain, when strength is equal to the uninjured side, and when the athlete is able to perform sport-specific activities (drills and skills associated with the sport) without pain.

Grade I sprains will usually take four to six weeks for the athlete to get back in the game. Grade II injury takes eight to ten weeks for full recovery, on average. Grade III injury takes about twelve to fourteen weeks to recover. Treatment of isolated MCL and LCL injuries does not require surgery. Conservative treatment is successful in most cases.

And then there's the ACL. It has been said that the three most frightening letters in the NFL are A-C-L. An injury to this ligament is very serious. In the past, a tear of the ACL would have been career ending. Now it is considered season ending.

The anterior cruciate ligament helps stabilize the knee by connecting the tibia (shinbone) to the back part of the femur (thighbone). This connection of the two bones keeps the shinbone from sliding forward in relationship to the thighbone. Usually, the ACL is a strong ligament and keeps the knee stable with cuts, twists, sudden stops, side-to-side motion, and pivoting.

In sports where there is stop-and-go activity such as basketball, tennis, football, and soccer, this ligament is a key stabilizer of the knee.

An injury to the ACL is much more common than to the PCL (posterior cruciate ligament) by about ten to one. The diagnosis of ligament injury may be by history and physical examination. MRI can be used to reinforce the diagnosis.

If there is a minimal or partial tear of the ACL with only a little instability, the athlete can avoid surgery and go forward with rehabilitation. A brace must be used for a return to play in most sports. A complete tear of the ACL with significant instability will usually require surgery to repair the ligament in order for the young athlete to return to play.

The timing of surgery in the younger athlete is important because kids have open growth plates. Special testing (bone age) must be done to see how much growth is remaining in the bones.

- If there is less than 1 cm of growth remaining, the athlete is treated as an adult. A reconstruction is recommended.
- If there is more than 1 cm of growth remaining, ACL reconstruction may not be recommended. A modified technique may be suggested and discussed with the sports medicine doctor.

The most commonly used technique for ACL reconstruction in kids uses a technique that minimizes the risk of growth disturbance, and surgeons have developed techniques to avoid growth plate injury. We can delay reconstruction until maturity is complete, but that might risk instability episodes and damage to the joint. I usually recommend reconstruction in order to reduce recurrent instability episodes and further damage to the joint.

An adult-type ACL reconstruction is usually done in females over age fifteen and males over sixteen. Otherwise, a graft is used to reconstruct the ACL and avoid hardware at the level of the growth plate. Any drill holes made to receive the graft should be small. With careful attention to surgical technique the ACL reconstruction in kids should be safe and effective.

If you are in this situation, talk with your surgeon and have him or her explain the options and the techniques. Ask questions about risk. Those are all fair points for discussion.

Return to play after an ACL reconstruction is a minimum of six months. The initial period following ACL surgery (reconstruction) uses a brace and rehabilitation. The athlete will progress to full weight bearing, exercises, weight training, and sport-specific drills and skills. When the athlete returns to play, especially in a contact sport, a brace is usually recommended.

Although female athletes have been known to be at increased risk for ACL injury, there are studies that indicate that neuromuscular training may help prevent these injuries. A study of female adolescent soccer players who participated in a fifteen-minute neuromuscular warm-up program twice a week showed they had a significant reduction in the rate of ACL injuries (Wilk et al. 1999).

This Swedish study looked at female soccer players who were twelve to seventeen years old. During the 2009 season, one group did the series of six warm-up exercises focused on knee control and core stability. One group did not do these warm-ups. The analysis of the data indicated a 64 percent reduction of ACL injuries in the group that did the neuromuscular warm-ups. The message here is that knee exercises are recommended, especially for girls in sports. They just might have fewer knee injuries.

Most ACL tears occur without direct contact. The injury occurs during sports such as soccer, volleyball, basketball, football, gymnastics, and skiing. Usually the player will state that he or she planted a foot and pivoted sharply. Injury also occurs when the player locks or extends the knee after jumping and lands on a straight leg and not a flexed knee. The extended knee mechanism may be more common in girls.

ACL injuries can also happen when the athlete stops suddenly or is clipped or hit from the side with the foot planted. This is a painful injury, and the player knows something serious has happened in most circumstances. The athlete will feel that the knee gave way and may have felt or heard a pop.

One female volleyball player described the feeling as the worst pain she had ever felt, as she landed on an extended knee after a block. She felt as if everyone around her must have heard the pop, and she thought she had broken her leg as she fell to the ground and grabbed her painful knee. I cringe every time I see a girl land on an extended knee or run in an upright, stiff position. They are just accidents waiting to happen.

It is hard to walk on the leg after an ACL tear. The knee will get swollen in a couple of hours along with severe pain with weight bearing and bending of the knee. The first two days are usually the worst, so if surgery is required, it may be postponed until the swelling has decreased. At the same time an ACL tear occurs, it is not unusual for there to be an injury to the cartilage (meniscus) of the knee.

Teenagers are a high-risk group for ACL injuries. This may simply be because they are more active. The highest-risk kids are those who play sports that involve cutting, pivoting, sudden stops and starts, and jumping.

Knee ligament injury statistics for females are consistent across high school, college, and Olympic levels. Ankle and knee injuries, along with calf injuries, rank highest for injury severity and lost playing time in females. Females suffer more lower limb injuries, while males suffer more facial injuries.

Females have a higher rate of serious knee injuries and are three to five times more likely to sustain an ACL injury when compared to males. Anatomical, hormonal, and biomechanical differences between females and males have been suggested as possible reasons why female athletes are more prone to sustain knee ligament injuries than male athletes.

Biomechanical testing of female basketball players, across all age groups, shows that the younger females tend to jump and land similar to boys until about puberty. The test was conducted by filming jumps off a plyometric box. The younger girls tend to land with their knees in alignment with their hips and ankles.

As the girls enter puberty, the knees start to fall into valgus (knock knees), placing more stress on the knee joint. This may be a result of the girls getting wider hips and attempting to keep their center of gravity and balance. It is very difficult to correct for this, even with rigorous training. However, strengthening the vastus medialis is a good exercise to help stabilize the knee in a female player. (The vastus medialis is the big muscle of the quadriceps on the inside of the thigh. Exercises such as squats and leg press on a machine can strengthen this muscle.)

Why Girls Get More ACL Injuries than Boys

- Girls, more than boys, use the ligaments more than their muscles to stabilize joints in sports.
- Boys, at puberty, increase in height and develop lower leg muscle strength (and mass) at the same time, but girls don't tend to develop lower extremity strength unless they strength train.
- Girls land with their legs in a more straight leg position (may be hip weakness) and cannot use their quadriceps muscles as shock absorbers as well as boys.
- Girls' knees tend to go into valgus (knock knee) when they are landing from a jump, pivoting, and side-to-side movements, and this position does not provide as much balance.

- Girls have wider hips and this may contribute to the knee position of valgus (looks like they are caving in), as the body keeps the center of gravity going down the center of the body (plumb line), which puts more stress on the ACL.
- Boys use their hamstrings (back of thigh muscles) while jumping and girls generally use their quadriceps (front of thigh) muscles, which pulls the shinbone (tibia) forward and puts more stress on the ACL.

Now you know. Can athletes, especially female athletes, do anything about the ACL vulnerability? Girls can't change their anatomy, but they can strengthen their legs.

Leg strength is less in female athletes, and they have slower muscle reaction times than males, which would increase the risk of injury. However, this is the one thing that can be corrected in females. Strengthen the muscles of the leg and the core muscles of the back, buttock, and abdomen, which keep the body upright.

The hamstrings need to be strong to keep the tibia in place during landings from jumps and sudden stops. In addition, the hamstrings help increase the speed with which girls react to ACL stressing movements. If female athletes react slowly, they are unable to protect their ACL. Women need to strengthen their hamstrings to protect their ACL.

Plyometric exercises and instruction on proper jumping technique are also important to prevent injury. Good examples of these exercises are tuck jumps, squat jumps, 180-degree jumps, ankle bounce, and broad jump. Girls need to learn how to "stick" their landings and hold the landing point for five seconds. Girls should avoid landing on an extended knee (more common in females) and land with the knee flexed.

We're not done with the knee yet. This is a complicated anatomical area.

Kneecap Pain

Pain behind the kneecap, called patellofemoral pain, affects around 10 percent of active adolescent girls, especially athletic girls. Kids with this problem will complain of pain while running, walking stairs, or performing other activities that involve repetitive weight bearing with a bent, or flexed, knee.

Commonly, the pain is in the middle of the kneecap. In the past, this knee pain was thought to be caused by girls having weak muscles in the thigh (vastus medialis) or overpronation (outside to inside roll of the foot like a flat foot). New research indicates that patellofemoral pain may be a product of hip weakness and poor control of the thighbone (femur) during weight-bearing activities such as sports.

In other words, poor mechanics in the leg and especially weakness in the core (abdominal and low back muscles) and hip area can lead to kneecap pain. It is thought that weak hip muscles cannot control the hip during weight bearing. Thus, the lower extremity will have poor mechanics with hips moving inward, creating knock knees.

Poor mechanics are easily seen during a single leg hop. Have your daughter try jumping on a single leg. See for yourself. The knee may cave inward, like a knock knee position. The girl should be able to stick the landing and hold that position for five seconds. The knock knee position during the landing, changes the relationship between the patella (kneecap) and the femur (thighbone) and increases joint stress.

Physical therapy can make big improvements in the poor mechanics. It is recommended that the athlete with this type of kneecap pain do stretches and strengthen the hip and the core muscles. A single leg squat is a simple test of lower extremity mechanics, hip strength, and injury risk (Carry et al. 2010).

Patella (kneecap) dislocations and subluxation (an incomplete dislocation) are also known as instability of the kneecap. There are two ways this injury occurs. One way is direct trauma to the kneecap, causing it to displace. Another way is indirect trauma associated with sudden slowing or stopping with a twist or change in position.

A complete dislocation will occur when the kneecap comes completely out of the joint (patellofemoral groove) and will usually go back into place by itself when the athlete straightens the knee. If the kneecap remains dislocated, the knee should be splinted, ice applied, and only a doctor should attempt to put the kneecap back in place (reduction). Athletes with subluxation (incomplete dislocation) may complain of their knee feeling as if it may give way.

Factors that may put an athlete at risk for kneecap problems are loose ligaments, flat feet, internally rotated hips, knock knees, or quadriceps weakness.

A doctor would need a medical history, physical examination, and x-rays to help make the proper diagnosis. PRICE MM is the initial treatment. Surgery is recommended if there is a large loose body (fracture fragment) floating in the knee joint that may cause further damage. Splinting in a straight position may be recommended for a period of time. There are functional patella braces that may help the player return to sports and feel more stable.

Recurrent dislocations and subluxation can be a big problem. Corrective surgery is considered if a rehab program has failed and full strength has been achieved in the quadriceps muscles.

Anterior knee pain (pain in the front of the knee) is a big problem. There are multiple causes of anterior knee pain including patellofemoral syndrome (kneecap pain), quadriceps and patellar tendinitis (jumper's knee), Osgood-Schlatter disease (an over use injury just below the knee), and iliotibial band syndrome.

Iliotibial band syndrome is one of the more common causes of pain on the outside of the knee in the running athlete. The band is a thick fascia on the outside of the knee that helps stabilize the knee during running. The rubbing of the band with flexion and extension may cause inflammation and pain on the outside of the knee. Usually stretching the iliotibial band helps this condition. A physical therapist can show the best way to stretch.

Don't get too stressed over the terms, which I'll quickly discuss, but do understand that the knee is a complex joint in a very complex limb (the leg). Lots of structures can be injured.

With knee pain in front, the problem is usually from overuse or doing too much activity too soon. In other words, the frequency, duration, or intensity of workouts may have increased too rapidly. This may cause the muscles to fatigue and lose their protective power and allow repetitive microtrauma to occur, which can lead to structural injury. Shoes and playing surface may also be a factor in overuse injuries.

Patellofemoral syndrome is a problem of the kneecap joint. Athletes with the "terrible triad" of flat feet, hip anteversion (hip rotates inward), and knock knees may be at risk for this problem. Obese kids are also at risk. The problem usually begins with poor position and tracking (the kneecap is not gliding in the right direction) of the kneecap or direct trauma to the kneecap causing injury to its articular surface.

The diagnosis is made by the history, physical examination, and x-rays. The athlete will usually complain of vague pain in the front of the knee and cannot point to the exact point of pain. The pain is behind the kneecap.

The usual treatment is PRICE MM. This is followed by aggressive lower extremity stretching and strengthening of the quadriceps (especially the VMO, vastus medialis muscle, on the inside of the thigh). Functional patella bracing can be helpful. Surgery is rarely required.

Jumper's Knee

Quadriceps and patellar tendinitis are both considered "jumper's knee." This injury is an inflammation of the quadriceps tendon where it inserts onto the top of the kneecap or the patella tendon and its insertion below the kneecap.

This is a true overuse injury most commonly seen in basketball and volleyball players because of the hard surface on which these sports are played and the intense jump training. The first line of treatment is PRICE MM. Quadriceps and patellar tendinitis will not get better unless there is rest and avoidance of jumping. Stretching and strengthening of the quadriceps is important for rehabilitation.

A well-cushioned athletic shoe will help prevent the pain from coming back. Knee straps may be used with some relief. If the athlete just plays through the pain, there is a risk for rupture of the tendon.

Osgood-Schlatter, Not Good at All

Osgood-Schlatter disease is not really a disease. It is an overuse injury that occurs where the patellar tendon attaches to the shinbone (tibia) in the lower leg. The site is actually a growth plate. Repetitive jumping and running can cause microfractures at the growth plate. The ongoing injury and repair cycle causes the characteristic bump under the kneecap.

The first treatment is PRICE MM. The athlete may have to stop the sport for some period of time in order to become pain free. In some severe cases, a cast may be necessary. When pain free, stretching and strengthening begins. If the athlete is pain free, he or she may return to sports. The end of growth brings closure to the growth plate and usually fixes this problem. Surgery is considered only if the resultant bump is painful. The bone spur is removed, and the problem usually goes away.

The entire body is a linkage system. At the very bottom of the human body are the foot and the ankle. They too can take a beating.

FEET AND ANKLES

Quick quiz: In which youth sport do you expect to see the most ankle sprains? Of course, basketball with 45 percent. Soccer accounts for another 31 percent of ankle sprains, and volleyball 25 percent (www.nata.org).

An ankle sprain is a ligament injury. You will recall that ligaments attach bone to bone and provide stability to a joint. An injury to the ligament is called a sprain. Earlier in this chapter I discussed the three grades of injury to a ligament from grade I as mild, grade II as moderate, and grade III as severe.

The most commonly injured ligaments are the lateral collateral ligaments of the ankle (the ligaments on the outside of the ankle). These ligaments are called the anterior talofibular ligament (the most commonly torn), the calcaneofibular ligament, and the posterior talofibular ligament. These ligaments can be injured when you "roll" over the outside of your ankle.

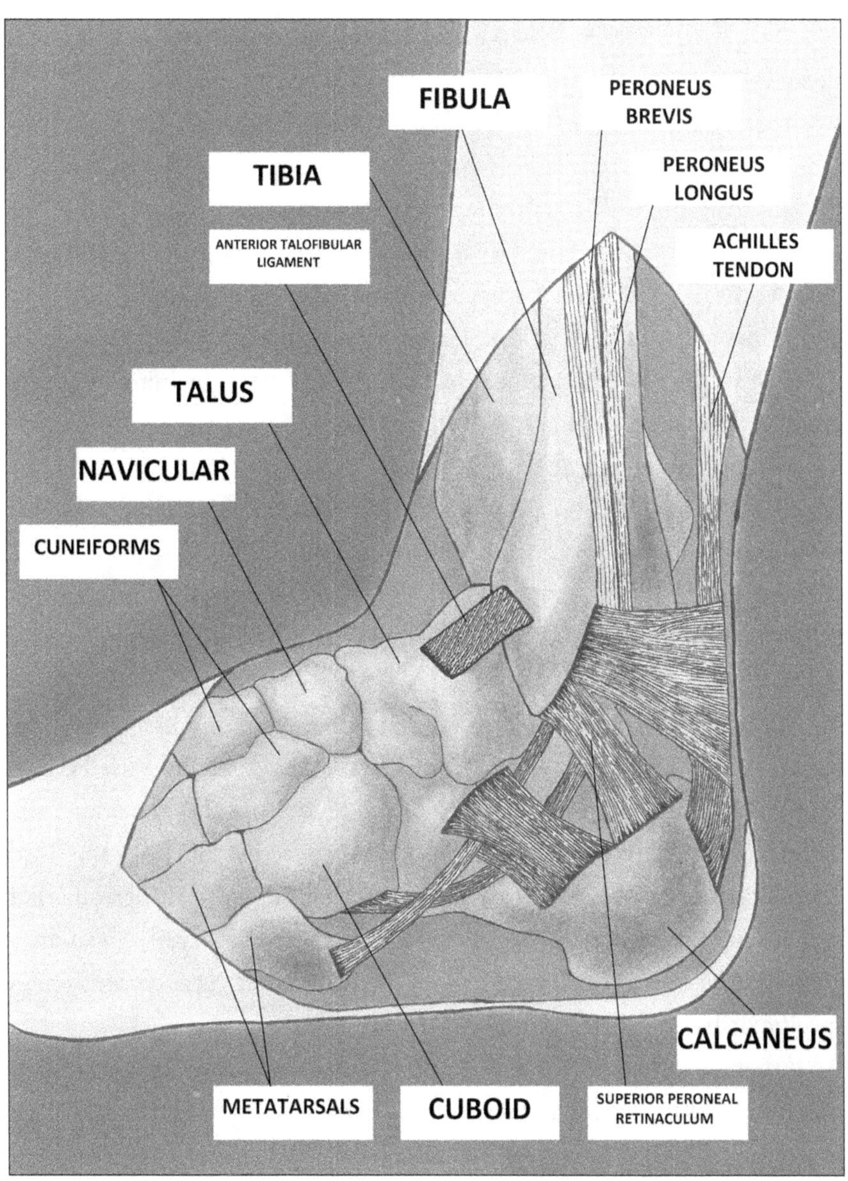

Anatomy of the Ankle.

Other structures can be injured at the time of the original injury. Bones of the ankle or the foot may fracture, a tendon can be torn or strained, and the nerves can stretch. Remember that an ankle sprain is not always "just a sprain." Several structures can be injured in one incident.

Usually, the athlete has a history of having his or her foot pointed down (plantar flexed) and inward (inversion). You can feel that motion now by simply pointing your foot down and inward. Then imagine you feeling you have rolled over the side of your ankle or foot. That's the mechanism at work here in creating an ankle sprain.

If this injury happens, the athlete may hear a pop or not have the ability to walk on the limb. It is important to find out if there is a history of a prior sprain or if this athlete has a "trick ankle." If the athlete heard a pop or was not able to put weight on the ankle after the injury, chances are that the injury was a grade II or grade III.

With a young player who is still growing, the growth plate on the outside of the ankle (fibula) may be injured and even require a cast. This should be evaluated by a doctor. Don't guess.

The goal of treatment is to prevent long-term problems, pain, or instability of the ankle. Rehabilitation is the key to avoiding future problems.

All ankle sprains are treated in three phases: In the first phase, the athlete will have the injury protected by tape or a brace and use PRICE MM. Stretching and strengthening of the tendons on the outside of the ankle and the Achilles tendon take place in the second phase. In the third phase of treatment, the athlete will try brisk walking or running and other maneuvers such as cutting or side-to-side slide. Then the athlete's balance and coordination are sharpened along with agility, endurance, and sport-specific drills.

Athletes with grades I and II injuries usually move quickly though the three phases. During phases two and three, grades I and II injuries are protected with tape and or a brace. Grade III injuries need to be protected with the ligaments in the proper position. This can be accomplished with a dorsiflexion (upward bending of the ankle) brace or a cast.

It is important that if a cast is used it is weight bearing as soon as the athlete can tolerate it. The cast is usually removed after about two weeks. The athlete is then advanced to phases two and three of treatment as tolerated. Surgery is not recommended in the early stages of ankle sprains.

A common location for an acute injury to the growth plate is the lower part of the fibula (this is the small bone on the outside of the ankle). The growth plate on the fibula may be injured after twisting the ankle or suffering an "ankle sprain."

Initially, this injury may be "walked off" by players and others and called "just a sprain." In this case, the injury is not taken seriously on the sidelines and not treated soon enough. The result, unfortunately, can be long-term problems such as the ankle giving way, a "trick ankle," or a weak ankle. Be aware of the "ankle sprain" that does not get better in about two weeks. It is not a minor injury that can be "walked off."

The lower part of the tibia (the big bone at the ankle), and lower part of the femur (the thighbone around the knee) may also have injuries to the growth plates. A proper history and physical examination will help make the correct diagnosis.

If the coach or trainer tapes the player for a sprain, it should be noted that tape restricts the extremes of motion and shortens the reaction time of the peroneal tendons, which protect the ankle. Also, nerve reaction time (called proprioception) may also improve with tape on. On the other hand, tape requires an experienced person to apply it correctly. It also loosens after about twenty minutes of play and should be reapplied.

Braces do not impede performance and are easier to apply than tape. Many braces are held on by either Velcro or laces and fit into a standard athletic shoe. High-top athletic shoes have been shown in some studies to decrease ankle sprains in basketball players. Braces have been shown to decrease ankle sprains in football players and female volleyball players. It should be pointed out, however, that no form of external support completely eliminates ankle sprains.

Bad Breaks

The most common foot and ankle fractures are to the ankle, heel, metatarsal (foot), toe, and sesamoid bones (twenty-six little bones in the foot). The diagnosis of a fracture is usually made by viewing the x-rays. Again, a fracture is a broken bone.

The treatment of a fracture is based on where it is located and how bad it is. In general, the best results will restore full function and use of the foot and ankle.

A Minilesson on Walking and Running

When walking or running, a person usually lands on the heel and then raises the heel off the ground, with the weight of the body moving forward onto the ball of the foot. The body is now ready to propel or push forward, and this maneuver is called "push-off."

The push comes off the ball of the foot, with much of this push-off coming from under the big toe. Weight is then shifted to the other foot.

The average person's stride length is 2.5 feet long. That means that for every mile that you walk, you take two thousand steps. If you are running, that is about fourteen hundred steps per mile. The longer your stride, the fewer steps you take.

Toes

Nothing can be more immediately painful than jamming or stubbing a toe. Most common injuries to the toes are fractures from jamming or stubbing the toes or when someone steps on the toes (volleyball and basketball are notorious for this) or drops an object on the toes (you being careless in the weight room).

It is rare for toe injuries to require surgery. The best remedy is usually just taping the injured toe and a stable shoe (one that does not bend easily) to heal. It usually takes four weeks for the toe to heal after a fracture. There are growth plates in the toes, and they are commonly the area where a fracture occurs, as is the case in other bones.

Injuries to the capsule and ligaments that hold the joints together can also occur. One injury is more common than others, and this is called "turf toe." Turf toe is a frequently used term that describes a sprain to the ligaments around the big toe joint. It is often associated with football but can occur in any sport and is seen in basketball, soccer, baseball, dance, gymnastics, and wrestling.

Turf toe occurs when a player has his or her foot in the push-off position and then another player lands on the back of the heel. It can also occur by jamming the big toe or repeatedly pushing off the big toe with force, during running or jumping. These are common mechanisms for this injury to occur, but any misplaced push-off type maneuver can cause this injury, in theory.

These maneuvers cause hyperflexion of the big toe, which gets pushed back more than is normal, and the ligaments are stretched or torn, resulting in turf toe. Typically this is a sudden injury and has been reported most often on artificial turf, which is why it is called turf toe. It can occur on any surface, especially if the athlete's shoes are worn down and are too flexible in the front part of the shoe under the ball of the foot.

The big toe works as a hinge for up and down motion, and the ligaments hold the bones of the hinge together. There are also two small bones on the bottom of the big toe, just behind the joint, called sesamoid bones—two small, pea-sized bones embedded in the tendons that move the toe downward. The sesamoids provide leverage for the tendon when you walk or run. The sesamoid bones can also be injured with a push-off injury.

How to tell if a kid has turf toe? Usually, the toe will hurt on the bottom of the foot, near the ball. The big toe may swell and become black and blue. If the pain is from repetitive motion and not one single injury, the symptoms may get worse over time. Sometimes when the injury occurs, a pop may be felt on the bottom of the big toe.

Turf toe is usually treated with a tape technique that limits full upward motion of the toe for about four to six weeks, and then an insert may be placed into the playing shoe. The insert should limit flexion of the big toe upward for about three months or to the end of the season, whichever is longer.

The doctor treating your child for turf toe should examine the athlete's shoes and make sure they are not too flexible or worn down. In some cases a cast and crutches may be recommended to rest the big toe and allow the tissues to heal. Some players will need physical therapy to regain full range of motion, as the toe may get stiff after the injury.

Occasionally, there may be a fracture of the small sesamoid bones on the bottom of the big toe. They are hard to see on x-rays but can create pain on the ball of the foot, under the big toe. Usually a pad can be placed into a stable shoe to protect the sesamoids for about three to six months.

If they continue to hurt after this period of time, an MRI may be ordered to get a three-dimensional image of the sesamoid bones and see if they are healing. If they are not, and they are painful after about six months, occasionally surgery is necessary to remove the injured bones. The surgery to remove the sesamoids is very rare in kids.

Achilles

The Achilles is a large tendon that crosses the back of the ankle and helps with push-off. The Achilles tendon inserts on the back of the heel bone. It is the most commonly injured tendon in the body. And it is a painful injury.

In the growing athlete, the Achilles tendon can become inflamed with tendinitis (tendinosis) and even cause problems at the point that it inserts into the calcaneus (heel bone). There is a growth plate in this location, and when it is pulled on by a tight Achilles tendon, the result is heel pain at the back of the heel. This has several names, but essentially it is called pediatric Achilles tendinitis. It has also been called apophysitis or Sever disease (discussed earlier under growth plate injuries).

The most common cause of Achilles tendon problems in athletic kids is a tight Achilles tendon. Either the Achilles is just tight because no stretching has been done, but also it can become relatively tight during a growth spurt when the long bones of the leg grow and thus put "stretch" on the Achilles tendon.

It is very rare for a young person to rupture the Achilles tendon. That's a special place for pain in adults.

SUPPORT: CASTS, BRACES, AND INSERTS

Casts: Casts are more often used in kids than for adults, especially if the growth plate is involved or there is a fracture. We orthopedic specialists use a cast to hold the leg or the arm in the proper position until healing is confirmed. The cast may be used for a broken bone, torn ligament, injured tendon or muscle, or even for skin healing.

In the past, plaster was used, but now fiberglass is the most common material. Fiberglass is lighter, dries much quicker than a plaster cast, and comes in every color. Several layers of cotton are wrapped around the arm or leg before the fiberglass goes on. The fiberglass looks like bandages and needs to be soaked in water before the layers are rolled on. The outer layer of fiberglass will be wrapped on the limb and then allowed to dry to a hard and protective coating.

For broken bones of the arm or leg, a child might wear a cast for around four weeks. Typically a cast is used for two to six weeks, depending on the injury.

We advise our kids to keep the cast dry. Fiberglass casts are water resistant, but the lining that is put underneath them is not. We can apply a waterproof liner, but it tends to not be as well padded. The doctor usually will decide if it is okay for your child to get a waterproof lining. Fiberglass casts with waterproof liners let the kid bathe, and even go swimming, during the healing phase. The liner that is waterproof and allows evaporation can only be used for certain types of fractures.

For the first twenty-four to seventy-two hours after a cast is placed on your child, it needs to be elevated. In other words, prop the arm on the arm of the couch or lift the casted leg in a recliner. Use pillows for propping in bed. This elevation prevents much swelling.

We also encourage kids to keep moving their toes and fingers to keep the circulation moving and also to avoid swelling.

Casts can get itchy. And a kid can't get to the itch. They can be miserable (and make parents miserable too). Don't stick anything into a cast. Try directing a hair dryer on a cold setting to blow down the cast.

Never put the hair dryer on a warm setting because it can heat up the fiberglass and burn the skin.

Sometimes ten minutes of ice above the itchy area can help with the misery. Occasionally an over-the-counter antihistamine can be used, but check with your doctor first.

I have pulled out all sorts of items from casts when they are removed from kids. This includes money, bugs, sticks, hair clips, food, toys, and homework!

Taking a bath or shower with a cast is nearly impossible, but kids can cover a cast on the arm with plastic bags and duct tape and try to keep the arm raised in the shower. If modesty is a problem, then a bath may be easier. For casts on the legs and feet, your kids just might have to have help washing.

Check your local pharmacy or drugstore for shower sleeves to put over a cast. They work like a heavier plastic bag with a Velcro cinch. No guarantees here; water has a way of getting into a cast.

If casts get wet, then call your doctor. The cast should be removed and changed to a clean/dry cast. If a wet cast remains in place, it can create an environment like a trench, and the skin may peel, become infected or necrotic, and require further treatment.

Taking off the cast seems scary, but it's not. The buzzing of the saw is really just vibrations and won't cut the skin. Most kids (and parents) are just relieved to get the darned thing off.

Braces: Common methods used to protect the ligaments of the ankle from injury include tape or an ankle brace. External support of the ankle is thought to provide mechanical stability, limit the range of motion, and improve nerve reaction time.

But even tape will fail after about twenty minutes of playing time or exercise, according to research (Pedowitz et al. 2008). And after an hour, athletic tape provides no significant support. In my view, tape is a poor option because teams just don't have the budget to buy tape, and athletic trainers don't have time to apply and reapply tape to protect ankles.

The best alternative is a brace, which is a device that is applied to help straighten or align a body part. It is used to protect the joint on which it is worn. Braces often restrict the extremes of motion of the joint. Athletes can put these on themselves and adjust them. Braces can, of course, be reused, which makes them a cost-effective option.

Wearing a knee brace may be useful in preventing ligament injuries (Verrone et al. 2000). There aren't many studies about how effective they are, but one study found that basketball players who wore an air stirrup brace had fewer ankle sprains than players who did not wear the braces (Sitler and Horodyski 1995).

Another study of soccer players found fewer ankle sprains among players who wore braces (3%) compared with players without a brace (11%) (Tropp et al. 1985). A brace may actually reduce the severity of the sprain and the incidence of reinjury for athletes who have a history of sprains.

What about athletes who are required to wear braces? A recent study looked at Division I NCAA female volleyball players who were required to wear double upright padded ankle braces (Pedowitz et al. 2008). During a seven-year period, the researchers studied athletes who wore the braces on both ankles and compared their injury rate with the injury rate for female NCAA volleyball players who did not wear braces during the same time period. Bottom line: The brace was found to be an effective way to decrease ankle injuries.

Watch Where You Land: Volleyball's Danger Zone for Injuries

Despite studies showing some benefit for volleyball players who wear ankle braces, protection from ankle sprains may depend more on the athlete's strength and conditioning rather than on the use of external support. However, the rigid and semirigid devices did appear to protect an ankle from an ankle sprain, to some extent. This was particularly true in the female players.

But volleyball has its own danger zone for ankle sprains. It's at the net. Here's why.

In volleyball, most of the ankle injuries occur at the net after blocking or attacking (Gross et al. 1994). Often the injured player has landed on the foot of an opponent or teammate. The blockers usually jump after the attacker, and since the attacker lands first, the blockers have an increased risk of landing on the foot of the attacker.

Under the net, the conflict zone is about twenty inches wide. That's where there's increased danger of landing on another player's foot. Since large forces are involved during landing after a vertical jump, especially onto another player's foot, the effect of bracing may be limited.

The main benefit of an ankle brace has been attributed to mechanical support. However, the large forces that are necessary to rupture a ligament may overcome any mechanical benefit provided by an external support. In other words, a player landing on your foot is much more powerful than any brace can withstand.

Volleyball, which involves continuous lateral movements and jumping, may even put more stress on the ankle than sports such as football, which involve intermittent activity. Perhaps this is why the ankle is more difficult to protect with external support in volleyball and basketball than in football.

A splint acts like a cast, but a splint can be removed. These can be made of leather or similar material and secured by Velcro closures that adjust for size and fit.

A splint is easier to remove and does not immobilize as well as a cast. A splint is usually used in the first stages of an injury, to allow for swelling. It can also be used at the last stages of an injury to allow for more motion.

A removable cast that has large Velcro straps to hold it on is not as good as a fiberglass cast for immobilization, but it is easy to apply, is removable for bathing, and allows walking.

I've discussed the acute injuries your kids may face in various sports. Of course, concussion must be taken seriously, but so should any strain or break or tear or rupture from head to toe. Acute injuries can happen in a flash. An elbow in the eye, a side swipe taking out a knee, an errant pitch to the head.

Another form of injury is the overuse injury, and I will tackle that next.

OVERUSE INJURIES

To put overuse injuries into perspective, imagine you're painting a fence. It's not a chore you do often, but in the spring you slap another coat on, repeating the brush strokes up and down, up and down, for the better part of a day. How is your shoulder going to feel the next day?

A little ice and maybe a Motrin, and in a few days you're fine. But if your child is throwing pitches or reaching overhead to spike volleyballs, day after day, with little rest in between, those shoulders are going to start screaming. Like your sore shoulder from painting, that's an overuse injury.

Medically, the overuse injuries to young athletes are caused by overload and repetitive microtrauma to the muscles and tendons of their immature skeletons. Like your shoulder pain from overuse in painting, early treatment of these injuries in kids is rest. If it hurts, stop doing it.

But it is often difficult to convince your child and the coach that rest is necessary (or the coach convincing a parent to let the kid sit out a while), especially in the face of a "normal" x-ray and a not-so-dramatic injury.

Every year, it seems that more kids participate in year-round sports. In addition, increased intensity and frequency of play lead to many young athletes developing overuse injuries. No longer are kids just practicing on a Saturday. They practice during the week and play on weekends. The play never takes a break.

In fact, overuse is responsible for about half of the sports injuries that happen to middle school and high school students. Overuse injuries usually occur over time with prolonged, repeated motion or impact. There is a range of overuse injuries that include muscle strains to more serious stress fractures (tiny cracks in the bone).

What Exactly Is an Overuse Injury?

Overuse injuries result from repetitive movements that put too much stress on the bones and soft tissues such as muscle and tendons. Mechanical stress from sports on the growth plate puts these growing areas at risk for injury. And remember, only kids, not adults, have growth plates.

Sports that require repeated loading such as baseball, basketball, football, soccer, rugby, tennis, gymnastics, and distance running may result in increased stress and injury to the growth plate. Most stress-related injuries do not upset growth.

In the past there have been some reports of growth plate injury from repeated stress in young gymnasts. Common sites for stress injuries to the growth plate are the knee (as takes place with Osgood-Schlatter disease), the heel (Sever's disease), and the elbow (Maffulli et al. 2011). One study noted that 38.3 percent of all acute growth plate injuries were sports related. Football was the sport with the highest risk to the growth plate.

Repetitive trauma (throwing pitches, running, hitting a volleyball overhead) produces microscopic cracking of the bone and produces pain. Continuing the activity that causes the pain causes more microscopic cracking at a rate that can be greater than the ability of the body to repair the cracks, resulting in a stress fracture.

This type of fracture is seen in the leg or foot of athletes involved in running sports such as cross-country. A special type of stress fracture that occurs almost exclusively in adolescents involves the lumbar spine. This condition, known as spondylolysis, produces chronic low back pain and is seen mostly in athletes who repeatedly hyperextend (bend backward) from their lower back, such as gymnasts and divers. See the earlier section on back injuries for more on this condition.

Any activity that involves repetitive motion, so common in sports, has the potential to cause an overuse injury. Kids participating in running, hitting, and throwing sports are especially prone to overuse injuries.

Sports involving throwing typically result in more overuse injuries to the shoulder and elbow. Running and jumping sports can cause more overuse to the lower extremity, causing such injuries as shin splints, tendinitis, or even stress fractures. The growth plate, as explained in the previous chapter, can suffer a stress fracture that is unique to growing kids.

Gymnastics, golf, and tennis can lead to overuse injuries of the hand, forearm, and wrist from gripping.

Poor training and conditioning can contribute to overuse injuries in student athletes. In addition to immature growing bones, not enough rest (or sleep) can contribute to an injury. In our survey of injured student athletes, we found that 33 percent got seven hours of sleep a night during the school week; 12 percent go nine hours; 9 percent got six hours or fewer; and 5 percent got ten hours of sleep. (The National Sleep Foundation recommends that teens get 9.25 hours of sleep per night to function correctly.) On weekends teens tend to get more sleep, with 23 percent getting nine hours; 16 percent getting eight hours; 14 percent getting seven hours; 12 percent getting six hours or fewer; and 7 percent getting twelve or more hours.

Sometimes an injured kid resumes training too soon, because the coach (or parent) tells the athlete to play through the pain. Commonly, the kid is anxious to get back on the field and doesn't report the pain.

Often it is not the return to play after the injury that is the problem, but rather the initial diagnosis of the injury. Youth sports injuries should be taken care of as soon as they happen. A doctor or trainer should evaluate every sports injury. Although overuse injuries are painful, most improve with rest. Ignoring any problem can turn it into a serious injury. Appropriate treatment and enough rest usually lead to recovery.

Causes of Overuse Injuries

- Growth spurts or an imbalance between flexibility and strength
- Poor or no warm-up period
- Too much activity (such as an increase in intensity, duration, or frequency of playing and training)
- Playing the same sport year-round or playing multiple sports during the same season
- Poor technique (such as overextending on a pitch)
- Poor equipment (such as worn-out or poorly fitting shoes)
- Poor playing surfaces (such as uneven field or slippery gym floor)
- Not listening to your child's body, especially pain
- Specializing too soon (at approximately thirteen years old or younger)
- Not enough sleep

When a child is growing, the bones grow quickly and may not be synchronized with the growth of the soft tissues, including the tendons and ligaments. If the bones have lengthened, this puts more stretch and stress on tendons and ligaments.

The bones that lengthen the most are the longest bones in the leg. These bones are the tibia and femur. The tendons and ligaments that attach to these bones get strained the most during growth, as the bones get longer. These tendons and ligaments are also at risk for overuse. The tendons attached to the long bones are the patellar tendon (which can cause jumper's knee, patellar tendinitis), and the Achilles tendon in the heel (Achilles tendinitis).

Weight training produces swelling and tightness of muscles and can make the problem worse, if not balanced by a proper stretching program. Even when coaches who recognize the importance of stretching prior to vigorous activity allow time for stretching in their practice schedule, young athletes may not be sufficiently aware of its importance and may loaf through stretching exercises. This puts them at increased risk for injury.

Lesson: Don't skip the stretching!

Education of young athletes as to the importance of stretching—as well as close supervision during stretching—may help prevent muscle injuries. Complete tendon ruptures are rare in the young athlete, fortunately. Most kids who have tendon injuries have a tendinitis, which is inflammation of a tendon, usually due to repetitive activity and overuse.

Appropriate treatment of tendinitis includes ice after activity, heat and stretching before activity, and modification or even stopping the sports activity.

COMMON TYPES OF OVERUSE INJURIES

Head to Toe: Shoulders First

Swimmer's shoulder is a general term which includes shoulder pain from overuse of the rotator cuff muscles and the muscles of the upper back. It is an inflammation and irritation of the shoulder caused by the repetitive overhead motion associated with swimming or throwing a ball (even though that is not swimming). The pain generally comes and goes at first. It may be possible to swim through the pain. The pain may progress to continuous. The child may even develop knots or painful points (trigger points) around the shoulder. The swimmer should work on developing a good symmetrical body rotation, bilateral breathing patterns, and avoid a thumb-first entry into the water. This will decrease the amount of stress and rotation of the shoulder.

Thrower's shoulder appears in kids who pitch. Studies have reported that there is an increasing rate of injuries and surgery to the shoulder and elbow in young pitchers (In Motion 2010). This may be from poor pitching form, overuse, and early introduction of the curveball. It may seem obvious, but kids who get injured in pitching tend to pitch more innings, throw more balls, and pitch more months in a year compared to other kids.

Baseball's governing bodies have reported an increase in injuries and have made rules to restrict the number of pitches thrown in a week (please see chapter 2 for a complete listing of the pitching rules).

Throwers' shoulders can become so loose and stretched out in the ligaments that the rotator cuff muscles cannot support the ball in the socket of the shoulder joint. This condition can occur in baseball, football, volleyball, softball, and track and field (shot put and javelin, for example).

Because the rotator cuff must now work overtime to attempt to support the joint, there is resulting inflammation and weakness. If the shoulder is not treated properly, a complete or partial tearing of the rotator cuff can occur and lead to surgery in some cases.

It is better to prevent thrower's shoulder than to treat it. The coach must not overwork throwing and overhead hitting athletes. It is of utmost importance that proper shoulder strengthening, conditioning, and throwing technique be instituted at a young age. Unfortunately, overworking the shoulder can create an injury no matter how careful the training program.

The nonoperative treatment for the shoulder that is injured includes PRICE MM. The young athlete must stop throwing (or hitting in volleyball) completely, become pain free, and then begin a strengthening program. Only when equal strength (to the opposite, uninjured shoulder) is restored can a program of hitting or throwing be resumed. Kids must rebuild their endurance slowly over time. Strengthening exercises must be continued for the remainder of the athlete's throwing career.

If practices such as rest, a short program of anti-inflammatory medication, and physical therapy over three to six months do not help the shoulder pain, an MRI may be needed to rule out a tear or significant injury to the ligaments or tendons around the shoulder. Shoulder instability or rotator cuff injury or both may require surgery to repair the injury. If the athlete returns to play, the coach should examine throwing and hitting mechanics and make corrections for improper technique.

Elbows

Like the overuse injuries for the shoulder, the elbow takes its share of abuse in throwing athletes too. And as in the shoulder, the forces around the elbow with overhead throwing and hitting sports are high.

Biomechanically, the throwing motion creates a significant force around the elbow in valgus (away from the body) movements. In other words, there is compression (squeezing) in the lateral (outside portion) aspect of the elbow and tension (stretching) placed on the medial (inside portion) of the elbow.

The more serious injury to the lateral (outside) of the elbow joint is called osteochondritis dessicans (OCD). We usually see these injuries in athletes thirteen to sixteen years old. It is common in baseball players and gymnasts.

The athlete will complain of pain and swelling in the lateral (outside) elbow that is worse with activity and has a loss of motion in the elbow joint. In cases that are not treated, there may be locking or catching in the elbow.

The diagnosis is made by a doctor taking a thorough medical history, physical examination, and x-rays (although they may be normal at first). The first line of treatment is ice, a splint, and possibly a sling for about four weeks. If caught early, the injury usually heals, and the athlete may return to play. However, this is a significant injury, and if there is a loose fragment of bone, surgery may be necessary in some cases. Usually we try about six months of nonoperative treatment first.

Injury to the medial (inside) side of the elbow is due to tension (stretching) that is placed on the elbow. This can cause inflammation of the growth site (apophysitis) and even a stress fracture of the growth area. If the pain progresses, the athlete will lose strength and distance. There may be swelling and decreased range of motion. The spectrum of these disorders is called "Little Leaguer's Elbow."

The first line of treatment usually includes six weeks of rest, ice, and anti-inflammatory medications. When the young athlete is pain free, he or she may gradually return to the overhead activity. But if the pain returns, the athlete usually is rested until the next season. Playing through the pain will make it worse.

Ligament injuries occur more often in older teen athletes. The ulnar collateral ligament (inside of the elbow) is more commonly injured in older adolescents and young adults. A complete tear of the ulnar collateral ligament usually occurs in the throwing athlete who complains of recurrent pain and swelling over the years.

The athlete may be pain free until returning to the throwing sport. This is usually followed by one event in which there is a "pop" in the elbow with significant pain as well as the inability to continue to throw. History, physical examination, x-rays, and an MRI are usually necessary to make the diagnosis. Surgery is often necessary.

Recommendations for Overuse Injuries among Young Pitchers

Added to the daily and weekly restrictions on young pitchers, it is also recommended that they do not pitch in competition or showcases for a minimum of four months of each year. Throwing that is not counted in a pitch count should also be limited, but is very hard to count. It is important that the young pitcher avoid excessive warm-ups and playing catcher.

If the elbow or shoulder is sore, there may be an injury. It is important for the athlete to report that soreness to the coach or parents. A good rule of thumb is if the adolescent pitcher requires anti-inflammatory medications, such as aspirin or ibuprofen, or needs to ice after each game, there is an injury that needs to be taken seriously, and the pitcher should rest. If the pain does not go away after a few days of rest, then the kid needs to see a doctor.

Knees and Below

One of the most common overuse injuries in the legs is Osgood-Schlatter disease. This disease usually occurs during the growth spurt in adolescence and especially in the athlete who is in a sport that involves repetitive bending and straightening of the knee, such as basketball and volleyball. It is most common in adolescents between the ages of nine and fourteen and is more likely among males than females.

Rapid growth spurts put a lot of stress on the insertion site of the patella tendon, where it inserts under the kneecap. Bone and tendon grow at different rates and are not always synchronized. The result? Periods of time when the tendon is relatively tight compared to the growing bone. You may hear the doctor call this the point where the patella tendon inserts on the tibial tubercle, which simply means an outgrowth of bone under the kneecap. It is a traction apophysitis and occurs at the upper area of the shinbone called the tibial tuberosity, a small lump under the kneecap.

So the whole mismatch puts traction and strain on the tendon. Osgood-Schlatter occurs more commonly in boys, with the greatest risk around thirteen years of age. There is pain, swelling, and tenderness just below the kneecap. The pain increases with direct pressure and with the knee fully extended (straightened) against resistance (in other words, if you try to straighten the knee and someone is pushing the opposite way against your leg to keep it from straightening) then there is more pain.

The treatment includes modifying the child's sports activities, relative rest, ice, and stretching and strengthening when appropriate. The focus of the stretching should be on the quadriceps, hamstrings, and iliotibial band.

Sometimes a brace, knee strap or tape will help. Usually this problem goes away over time. However, some pain may be present until the growth area of the bone (apophysitis) stops growing. About 10 percent of kids with this problem will have some discomfort in that area as an adult (and even a separate bone particle) (Wells and Sehgal 2011).

A commonly injured growth plate from overuse is the one on the back of the heel bone called the calcaneus. Overuse injury here can lead to pain at the back part of the heel and is seen in growing children, especially those engaged in running sports. This problem is often seen with a tight Achilles tendon. This problem is sometimes referred to as Sever's disease, but it is not a disease. It is an overuse problem.

Soccer may be a big offender here. This injury may be related to a negative heel—or a shoe that tilts backward and puts more stress on the heel. To see if the child's shoe is the problem, put the shoe on a flat surface such as a table (just the shoe, not the shoe with the kid in it!).

Check to see if the heel is lower than the toe area of the shoe. The negative heel will put more stretch on the Achilles tendon and can lead to overuse problems. The growth plate of the heel bone can also have more stress on it from a negative heel.

Only about 25 percent of soccer shoes have a negative heel. But if a child suffers from heel pain, do not let your child wear a shoe with a negative heel. As a matter of fact, a heel lift should be added to the shoe to decrease the stress on the Achilles tendon and the growth plate in the heel.

Treatment for this type of injury is usually quite successful. Sometimes physical therapy is recommended, and the kid should start a good stretching program. The Achilles tendon should be stretched. Anti-inflammatories can be used for a limited time, as directed by a doctor. If these simple treatments do not work, than the kid may need a cast. If the problem is not solved (and the pain gone), then an MRI is sometimes necessary. This problem is not treated with surgery.

HOW TO PREVENT OVERUSE INJURIES

Some sports are just not age appropriate. Throwing sports should be introduced after a kid has developed good coordination and balance. It's wrong to expect little boys and girls to pitch, for example.

That's the best reason for kids to play "coach pitch" until they are about seven years old and not try to advance faster through the baseball league—no matter what dad says about his "star pitcher."

The American Academy of Pediatrics has recommended that children not play any team sport until they are at least six years old. That recommendation seems strict, but it certainly sends the message, however, that advancing too fast too soon could lead to burnout and overuse injuries.

All kids who play sports can develop an overuse injury, but the likelihood increases with the amount of time a child spends doing an activity. A variety of activities is recommended to avoid overuse. For example, pitch counts (baseball) and limitation of the young athlete throwing (football) or overhead hitting (volleyball) can help. Since it is almost impossible to count throws and hits (aside from pitch counts), time in or rotation may be used to avoid overuse.

If a child has pain while doing any activity, it is causing damage to the body. A little soreness after the activity is fine, but even soreness can be a problem if it does not go away with about twenty-four hours of rest.

In coming off a period of relative inactivity, such as summer vacation, or after a change from one sport to another, a young athlete is at risk for overuse injury. These problems may be made worse by the limited time periods for training prior to the start of the season. It is actually more likely that this type of injury occurs as a result of the increasing demand on the body too rapidly rather than placing demands that would be considered excessive.

Although they are not completely preventable, overuse injuries can be minimized by cross-training, by education of the young athlete about preseason conditioning, and by carefully prepared training schedules (not too much too soon).

Discouraging early specialization may be a factor in avoiding overuse injuries. This is a decision the kid must make with his parents and coach.

Recommendations to Avoid Overuse Injuries

- Before your child begins a sport, get him or her into shape. Conditioning may include stretching, warm-ups, and aerobic exercise. These warm-ups are typically done on the field under the guidance of the coach. Prepare for activity with warm-up exercises and end with cool-down exercises—also done with the team.

- Children should get a physical examination every year while playing sports. Most sports programs require a medical clearance package to be filled out before your kid can play. Insist on a thorough physical exam, not just a quick look.
- Start your kid out slowly with a new sport and increase the training program and activity gradually. Again, this is better advice for the coach, but parents should be observant.
- Let your child take some time off from playing if he or she feels tired or is in pain. There is no point in overdoing it.
- Make sure the coaches stress the importance of the kids staying well hydrated by drinking enough water or even sports drinks (especially in hot weather). If your child feels hungry, tired, or thirsty, do not let him or her start practice or a game until those issues are addressed. Dehydration and hunger can cause fatigue and increase the chance of injury.
- Student athletes should wear athletic shoes that fit well and are in good condition. If your child participates in a sports practice or event three or more times a week, the kid needs sport-specific shoes. Sport-specific shoes should be worn for running, basketball, tennis, soccer, baseball, and football. Some sports have shoe requirements that are considered part of the "equipment," such as cleats for football, soccer, and baseball. Basketball shoes have specific features that give more control for side-to-side motion and sudden stops. Sprinters' shoes are lighter weight and more flexible than training shoes for running.
- If your child is injured, seek medical care right away.
- Injury prevention does not mean that your kids need to avoid sports and recreational activities. Even when injured, there are usually some exercises they can do such as weight training or riding a stationary bike.

TOO SOON: PLAYING AGAIN AND RISKING REINJURY

Quite simply, reinjury occurs when an athlete returns to play before he or she is fully recovered from a previous injury.

If an athlete returns to sports too soon, more stress is placed on the injured body part. A reinjury can occur during this time—with serious consequences. Other body parts, including the surrounding joints, are forced to make up for the injured joint and can also get injured. This is a common event, which may lead the young athlete into believing he or she is breaking down or becoming fragile. Reinjury is not good for the body and is horrible for player confidence.

Too early of a return to play is the most common cause of reinjury. The kid should reenter the sport gradually and in stages. The treating doctor should explain a sensible return-to-play program and schedule and write the plan down for the athlete (and the coach and parents). Of course, the injured athlete is usually eager to rejoin the team. But, as I tell my patients, missing a few games is better than coming back to see me.

"When can I get back in the game, Coach?"

The clearance for a child to return to play often falls on the doctor. And it should. Why? Because we are qualified to determine if the previous injury is healed and if the child has fully recovered.

To go against medical advice is risking a serious reinjury and all the disappointment that comes with missing the rest of the season or dropping off the team.

When I am asked how long healing will take, I can only go by averages for similar injuries. The average time for recovery after an ankle sprain, for example, depends on how bad the injury was.

A minor sprain (grade I) may take one week to recover. A moderate sprain (grade II) may take two to six weeks to recover. A severe sprain (grade III, and a complete tear of the ligaments around the ankle) may take from six to twelve weeks to recover completely.

When the player has been treated for the sprain, he or she should have full range of motion. When the athlete returns to play after an ankle sprain or ligament tear, a semi-rigid ankle brace or tape should be used for practice and games for six months or until the end of the season, whichever is longer. It is important to warm up, stretch the part, and strengthen the injured limb.

Every patient heals differently over time. Don't press your doctor to release your child before all indications are that the injury is fully healed.

I have observed reinjury many times, and it's heartbreaking. Once a kid has had more than one injury to the same body part, he or she begins to lose confidence—a tragic consequence for a young athlete.

It is important to make sure that the child has rehabilitated the injury before returning to sports. The athlete also needs to wear appropriate protective gear for the body part that was injured. This may be in the form of a brace or tape.

After a reinjury the young athlete must continue to maintain flexibility and strength in the injured area for the rest of his or her athletic career. I cannot stress this point enough. It is important to regain full range of motion and strength of an injured joint before returning to play. Confidence returns after a successful return to play without pain.

In a recent survey, we asked injured student athletes if they were pressured to play before they were ready, and 42 percent said yes. Of that group, 51 percent said that the pressure came from other teammates, 32 percent from their coaches, 4 percent from their parents, 4 percent from other school faculty, and 9 percent from others.

In the same survey, when asked how worried they were about having another injury after they returned to play, 40 percent of the injured young athletes were equally worried as before their injury; 30 percent said they were more worried about having another injury; 23 percent said they were less concerned about another injury, and 7 percent were unsure.

Of interest, 28 percent felt they were a better player after they returned to play after their injury; 40 percent thought they were the same; 21 percent thought they were worse; and 12 percent were not sure.

MY MEDICAL ADVICE

Compared to a decade ago, there are about three million more high school athletes. However, the injury rate has increased 500 to 700 percent. The increase in injuries may certainly be the result of more kids participating in sports, but also kids are playing like their heroes—professional athletes.

There is more money being invested in kids' sports than ever before. It has become a billion-dollar industry that is fed by more kids participating more intensely in their sport. They need more equipment, better equipment, the latest equipment, trainers, sport-specific trainers, and in many cases sports psychologists to teach "sports" mental toughness.

An unfortunate trend is that young athletes are specializing earlier than ever. Coaches, parents, and the players often think that they must focus on one sport and a set of skills as much and as soon as possible.

Kids are being recruited for elite club sports at record numbers. So perhaps they are playing harder and tougher. But also, injuries are being tracked and recorded better than ever. In addition, there is more awareness of many injuries, such as pediatric knee injuries and concussions. All of these factors contribute to the increase in injury rates.

My advice for kids to avoid early burnout and injury is not to specialize too soon. Do not allow your child to specialize until he or she is about fourteen. Specializing too soon will lead to overuse and burnout at an early age. Even a year-round sport should have at least three months of rest from the sport. That does not mean the student athlete gets out of shape; he or she simply changes it up and stops doing repetitive activity.

Kids should experience as many sports as they can. They may be good at pitching, but they also may be good at golf or cross-country or football. There is good evidence that they should not specialize until the senior year in high school. It is interesting to note that a high percentage of NBA players played more than one sport in high school, according to ESPN's *Behind the Lines.*

After an injury, practice should resume before competition. The game schedule should not influence the timetable for the athlete's return to play, even if the team is in the finals. Especially if the team is in the finals.

Listen to the child. If a child begins complaining of pain, it's the body's way of stating there is a problem. A doctor can usually diagnose many of these conditions by taking a medical history, examining the child, and ordering some routine tests.

It's important to get all injuries, including overuse injuries, diagnosed and treated to prevent them from developing into long-term problems. The doctor may recommend that the child temporarily modify or eliminate an activity to limit stress on the body.

As a team doctor, I know it's a challenge dealing with the parents and the kid with an injury. Both want to get back in the game sooner than is usually recommended. There are four *P*s that help in making decisions about a kid's sports injury and treatment: physician, patient, parent, and pain (thanks to Champ Baker, former AOSSM president).

All four need to be considered, but the pain and the physician know best. Pain can be useful. It will tell you when your child is hurt. Listen to the body.

In some cases, the kid may not be able to return to a sport without risking further injury. The doctor may advise rest, medications to help reduce inflammation, and physical therapy. Depending on the area that is injured, if the pain does not go away, a special test such as an MRI may be recommended. When recovery is complete, your child's technique or training program may need to be changed to prevent the injury from flaring up again.

Kids should not be pushed to play through pain—any pain, anywhere. A kid may not actually know when he or she is having pain or is just sore. If a kid starts to limp, avoids running, favors one side, asks for ice or anti-inflammatories or to come out of the game, the pain is significant. If the pain does not go away with twenty-four to forty-eight hours of rest, a doctor should be notified. Healing time can be shortened as soon as the injury is identified and treatment started.

4

You Throw Like a Girl: Understanding the Female Athlete's Injuries

With greater numbers of girls participating in sports has come an increased understanding of injuries and problems associated with the young female athlete. It is important for the coach, trainer, parent, and athlete herself to be aware of the specific risks that girls face playing sports.

Quite simply, girls are different. Physiological and sociological factors make the female athlete different.

On a social level, the image of a strong and fierce female athlete has evolved over several generations. Although the rough-and-tumble nature of sports has become more accepted for girls, the media bombard girls with the perception that they also need to maintain a supermodel stick figure and feminine, dainty ways. These conflicting signals create significant stress for some girls that leads to eating disorders and a serious disorder called the female triad, which I discuss in detail in this chapter.

Physiologically, the female athlete has to deal with menstruation and hormone balance. Stress, diet, overeating, not eating, overtraining, and other factors can alter the normal menstrual cycle and hormonal balance, which can lead to injury.

Now add to that some gender-specific differences in the musculoskeletal system. In other words, girls' bodies are different, too.

Here's the anatomy lesson: Women have wider hips than men, which create a wider angle at the knee, where the kneecap (patella) meets the femur (bone in the upper thigh). This increased angle (often called the

"Q-angle") affects the gliding (tracking) of the patella and predisposes the female athlete to tracking problems.

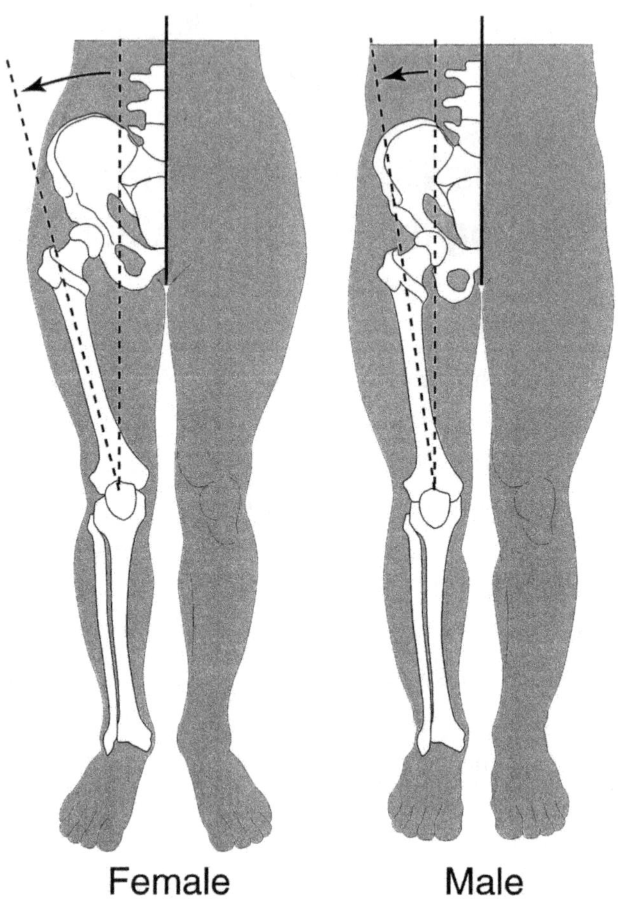

Female and Male Anatomy Differences. Females have a wider pelvis than males and a larger Q-angle at the knee. The Q-angle is the angle that the thighbone (femur) makes in relationship to the knee and hip (women appear more "knock kneed"). This may put more stress on the ligament, so the knee can become injured when cutting or landing from a jump in females. When the knees come closer together, this is called valgus. Women may roll in at the ankles more than men. That is called pronation.

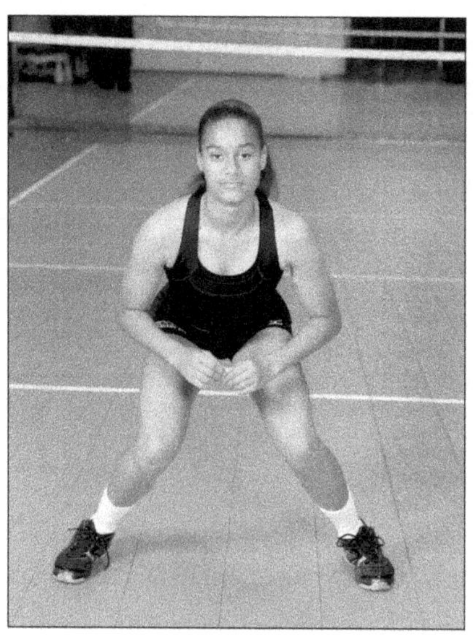

A

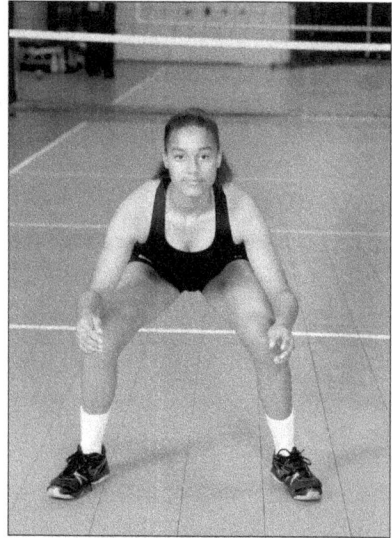

B

Knee Position: While performing jumps, lifts, or other leg exercises, sometimes it is easy to see the knee move into valgus (or cave in) (A). This can put the knee at risk for injury. This is more common in girls and can make them prone to knee injury. The knees should be centered over the foot to put less stress on the knee (B).

Abnormal tracking of the kneecaps may lead to instability or dislocation of the patella, or simply pain due to abnormal mechanics. Think of this as a tire out of alignment, where unbalanced loads lead to the treads wearing out on one side of the tire. A similar process is going on under the kneecap.

The young female athlete should emphasize strengthening exercises that help to improve stability of the knee, kneecap tracking, and injury prevention. These exercises should focus on the inner quadriceps (thigh) muscles (vastus medialis oblique or VMO).

The female athlete seems to be more at risk for injury to the major knee stabilizer, the anterior cruciate ligament (ACL). Why? For one reason, females tend to have a narrower space, notch, in the knee available for this ligament, so less stress is required to tear the ligament than in the male athlete.

Recent studies have shown that female athletes tend to rely on their quadriceps more than on their hamstrings as compared to male athletes. Since the hamstring muscles are one of the main protectors of the ACL, relative weakness in this structure may lead to ACL injuries.

Additional risk of injury may be related to estrogen levels. Female athletes tend to sustain injury to their ACL at the point in their menstrual cycle when they are ovulating (days 10–14). Estrogen levels are at their highest during this period. Studies show that the ACL contains estrogen receptors and that the ACL responds to estrogen by decreasing cell activity and production of the basic ligament fibers (collagen).

Preseason and in-season strength and conditioning programs that build knee muscle strength, particularly for the hamstrings, may help reduce the risk of injury.

Female athletes have been shown to have a higher incidence of ankle sprains than males. The higher number of ankle sprains in girls may be due to increased ligament laxity and decreased muscle strength and coordination compared to boys.

Strengthening and coordination exercises for the ankle are recommended to limit the risk of ankle sprains. Use of a balance board and elastic band exercises for inversion (turn-in) and eversion (turn-out) are helpful.

GIRLS ARE STRONG BUT NOT AS STRONG AS BOYS

As a group, girls are not as strong as boys. Upper extremity strength is 50 to 75 percent that of boys. Lower extremity strength is 60 to 80 percent of boys' strength in the legs. Studies have shown that, with weight training, females will increase their strength with percentage gains that are equal to males' but that their overall strength will begin and end at lower levels than boys. Due to lower testosterone in girls, the size of muscles will not increase as much as it will in boys.

Leg length in girls is a smaller percentage of overall body length than in boys and may be one reason that females tend to be slower runners than males.

Women seem to be catching up to men in endurance sports such as long distance running and swimming much more rapidly than in strength or speed events such as sprints. It is possible that women may in fact be more suited physiologically to endurance activity than men, due to an improved ability to conserve muscle glycogen (sugar used for energy) and ability to utilize fat for energy.

However, girls have a lower oxygen-carrying capacity, lower blood volume, fewer red blood cells (that carry oxygen), lower blood count (hemoglobin), smaller heart, and lower stroke volume (amount of blood pushed with each heartbeat), preventing them from obtaining performance levels equal to boys.

SURPRISING WAYS GIRLS ARE DIFFERENT

Girls are different from boys in many ways. Parents of teens know these distinctions well. But here we'll talk about some of the ways the female anatomy affects their play and injury. You may not be aware of some of these differences.

Females tend to have more lax ligaments than males, which is thought to put their joints at increased risk for injury. The risk of injury in females may correlate to hormonal changes associated with the menstrual cycle. In particular, girls may be more prone to knee ligament injuries, shoulder instability, and ankle sprains.

More girls get leg pain commonly known as shin splints. Shin splints are not a single medical condition. They can be simply a symptom of an underlying problem such as a stress fracture of the shinbone (tibia) or a mechanical problem such as flat feet or overpronation that puts more stress on the muscles, tendons, and bone of the shin. Another problem that can cause shin splints is swollen, irritated muscles.

In the orthopedic world, we call it exertional compartment syndrome, so tuck that term away in case you need it. This form of shin splints occurs only during exercise and quickly goes away after activity stops. The legs will tend to feel tight or swollen, especially while running.

In female athletes, menstrual cycle and use of birth control pills can affect fluid shifts in the muscles. In female athletes suspected of having exertional compartment syndrome, modification of birth control medication may solve the problem. This modification would include a change in dose or stopping altogether.

Scoliosis is a curvature of the spine that occurs in growing kids and is much more common in girls than boys. In the early stages of scoliosis, there are usually no symptoms. We often diagnose this in the female athlete who appears to have a difference in shoulder or pelvic height. Small spinal curves will not stop a girl from playing sports, but she should be seen by a doctor and watched for possible worsening of the deformity.

The younger female gymnast, ballerina, and jumping athlete (volleyball, basketball) are at risk for developing a spinal injury called spondylolysis. This is a stress fracture of the back, and I discussed it in an earlier chapter.

This injury is thought to result from the repetitive hyperextension (bending backward) required in these sports. Many of these girls are also not having their period (or periods are irregular), making them more prone to develop stress fractures. The at-risk female athlete with long-term back pain should be seen by a doctor and have x-rays to evaluate the situation.

WHAT TO CHECK IN A PRESEASON SPORTS PHYSICAL

In addition to the usual heart and other health issues to be checked in a preparticipation physical examination, female athletes need to be evaluated for certain problems specific to girls.

Scoliosis: Curvature of the spine is much more common in females and tends to occur in adolescence. During the preseason examination, your doctor should include a check for curvature of the spine, and, if present or suspected, x-rays and referral to a specialist may be recommended.

A change in posture or a difference in shoulder height or hip height should raise concern and should be evaluated by a doctor.

Scoliosis evaluation begins with a history and physical examination. The physical examination includes a forward-bending test. This test has the girl bend forward at the waist, with the arms hanging loose with palms touching. The doctor visually checks for a curve of the spine and an uneven back and ribs.

If the bone age (growing bones) is young, the risk for the curve getting worse is high. Scoliosis is often hereditary, and if someone else in the family has it, your daughter should be checked regularly. Scoliosis usually becomes apparent during puberty and the early teenage years. An x-ray can be used to measure the size of the curve.

Girls are more at risk for having hereditary scoliosis from their mothers. Scoliosis, if untreated and more severe, can lead to a hunch back and problems with breathing. If diagnosed early in the growing child, treatment is very successful. Once growing has stopped, the deformity is hard to correct.

Mitral valve prolapse: A common and usually harmless problem with the heart valves is mitral valve prolapse, which occurs mostly in females. With mitral valve prolapse, a very specific type of murmur (heart sound) can be found on the preseason heart check as the doctor listens with a stethoscope. Most cases have no symptoms and will not prevent sports participation. A heart specialist should see athletes with a history of fainting, irregular heartbeat, chest pain, or family history of heart disease.

Be sure your child's doctor knows the family history for not only heart issues but any other conditions. It just makes diagnosis so much more accurate and early. And knowing a family history of any condition raises the bar of suspicion in case your child is showing early signs that should not be ignored. It's always easier and smarter to treat a condition earlier rather than later.

Menstruation: The preseason physical for girls should include a menstrual history. The doctor will ask your daughter when her periods began. You'll want to make note of it too because this is an important date for lots of hormonal reasons (and injury prevention). Delayed onset of menstruation should be noted and may indicate possible eating disorders (and I'll get to that soon).

Ligament laxity: Females with excessive laxity (looseness) of their ligaments should be told that they may be at increased risk of knee, shoulder, and ankle injuries and should be encouraged to participate in preseason strengthening exercises to protect the joints. Girls are more flexible than boys at any age (Breighton 1973).

Increased looseness in the shoulder may lead to shoulder instability. Girls tend to have decreased upper body strength compared to boys, which may also add to the risk.

Girls with very loose kneecaps (patella) might be discouraged from running and twisting-type sports such as basketball. The kneecap dislocation occurs when the patella moves or slides out of place. The abnormal movement of the kneecap is usually toward the outside of the leg. Kneecap dislocations are most often seen in girls, usually after a sudden change in direction with the leg planted on the ground. This maneuver is seen in basketball, volleyball, and tennis. Girls with this problem will show a "sloppy" kneecap that slides around easily (the condition is called hypermobile).

In sports with overhead movements such as volleyball, tennis, swimming, and softball, shoulder laxity may be a problem. If a girl has very lax shoulders (loose shoulders), she might be told not to participate in swimming or volleyball.

However, I am reluctant to restrict the patient unless she has had a significant episode or problem with the shoulder. Some shoulder looseness is a result of adaptation such as the pitcher with increased rotation more than other players on the team. Elite-level swimmers also will develop more rotation and apparent looseness in the shoulder.

Shoulder instability is abnormal and can lead to pain, partial dislocation (subluxation), or dislocation. We see the condition in certain sports and sports positions such as pitcher in softball, outside hitter in volleyball, and elite swimming. It is very likely that these girls have already discovered that these positions and sports are painful on their shoulders.

Strengthening exercises may help prevent this injury. Internal and external rotation exercises using elastic tubes or bands can help. A trainer or physical therapist can show your daughter how to do these exercises.

Feet and toes: Girls tend to get bunions and hammertoes more often than boys (by a whopping ratio of nine to one). This may be genetic in some cases (if mom has bunions, her daughter may be at higher risk) but is more likely from wearing narrow shoes—only 10 percent of bunions can be attributed to genetics.

Bunions and hammertoes can be painful and affect athletic performance. Wider athletic shoes and bunion pads may be helpful. Improved shoe wear off the field may help prevent this problem. Kids seem to be wearing flip-flops these days for casual and even dress, in school and everywhere else. Frankly, they may be the best choice.

Wearing flip-flops (with a small arch, not the Brazilian flat ones) will allow the small muscles of the feet to contract and strengthen. This will result in stronger feet and fewer bunions and hammertoes. Flip-flops have also been shown to decrease the load that is translated to the knee when walking. So if your athlete (male or female) has knee pain, it is possible that wearing flip-flops will help decrease that pain.

Of note, the barefoot runners of the world tend to have fewer foot problems than the shoe-wearing runners. They have stronger feet and tend to run more on the midfoot and forefoot area. It is recommended that to begin a barefoot running program, ease into it and make sure that the feet are biomechanically sound (no bone and joint problems).

THE FEMALE TRIAD: EATING DISORDERS, AMENORRHEA, AND OSTEOPOROSIS

Here's a typical scenario. Your daughter is a gymnast or a swimmer. Maybe a runner. You notice her skipping family meals. She hides energy bars in her desk drawer. Her skin seems dry, and she's always putting a big baggy sweatshirt on because she's cold and because she's hiding a dramatic loss of weight. And that shoulder injury seems to be taking a long time to heal.

Now that's an extreme example of the female athlete triad, but it contains many of the common behaviors and symptoms parents and coaches should never overlook or explain away as a training issue or "just being a growing teenager."

By the time I see this girl in my office for an ankle fracture, she already has osteoporosis from thinning of bone and an increased risk of bone fractures. The fractures that are seen in the girls with the triad are usually stress fractures. The stress fracture is a microfracture in bone that results from repetitive load.

The common sites for these microfractures are the metatarsals (small bones of the foot), tibia (shinbone), and fibula (ankle bone on the outside). The contributing factors that can lead to these fractures are an increase in training volume or intensity; inadequate time to recover between training sessions; biomechanical problems such as a leg length difference; poor flexibility; muscle imbalance/muscle weakness, mostly in the calf; problem with alignment of the legs or feet; high arches; flat feet (yes, both of them); worn-out shoes or poor fit or design of the shoes; hard playing surface; poor diet; and, most importantly, the female triad. All these factors may exist or only some.

Fractures in these girls may at first go unnoticed because the bone fracture may not show up on x-rays for up to six weeks after the pain starts. A bone scan can be used to see these fractures early on. When the athlete has gotten to the point that the bone is breaking, she needs to reduce exercise and training to moderate levels. Strenuous and excessive training must stop until the dietary and hormone problems are improved.

The female triad consists of eating disorders, the stopping or irregularity of the menstrual cycle, and a dangerous decrease in bone density. This condition is serious and must be taken seriously. It won't go away on its own. Girls don't outgrow it. In fact, the condition worsens into adulthood and can cause lifelong problems. And if that isn't enough to scare a parent into taking action, let me add that a girl with one of these issues probably has the others going on too.

So let's look at the female triad and the individual health risks.

Eating disorders: Eating disorders are more common in sports where appearance is highlighted, such as gymnastics, figure skating, and diving.

The severity ranges from occasional binge eating to extreme self-starvation (this condition is called anorexia nervosa) and prolonged binge eating and purging or vomiting (the condition known as bulimia).

Depending on the studies we track, eating disorders may affect anywhere from 15 percent to 62 percent of female athletes (CDC, "Mental Health Surveillance"; The Renfrew Center Foundation for Eating Disorders 2003; Zucker et al. 1999; Sungot-Borgen and Torstveit 2004; Bachner-Melman et al. 2006). Parents, coaches, and trainers should be alert to behaviors that may signal a girl has an eating disorder. Does your daughter eat alone or push food around her plate but not really eat it? Does she make trips to the bathroom during or after meals to vomit the meal? Does she use laxatives?

Other signs or symptoms of the female athlete triad may include fatigue (your daughter is tired all the time, sleeps in), anemia (low iron but can only be determined by a blood test), depression (hard to diagnose in a teen, may shun friends, angers easily), cold intolerance (always wearing a sweatshirt or long sleeves even on hot days), and eroded tooth enamel (from frequent vomiting, which is something the dentist or dental hygienist might notice first).

You should be concerned if your daughter or player demonstrates an unreasonable fear of being fat, has a distorted sense of body image, or fails to maintain body weight within 15 percent of the mean for her age and height. Such an athlete might spend time in front of the mirror, talk too much about food or how "fat" she is, or constantly weigh herself or exercise to an extreme.

Anorexic athletes show extreme weight loss (and they may seem happy about it), but at the same time, their body systems are being irreparably harmed. The heart takes a hit, as do the endocrine and gastrointestinal systems. Hormone balances are off. Bones are not building; they are breaking down (a warning sign is a female athlete with fractures).

Sadly, all these issues can lead to death. The mortality rate in severe cases is particularly high at 10 to 15 percent with death occurring primarily due to cardiovascular failure, endocrine disturbances, or suicide.

The bulimic athlete engages in binge eating and forces herself to vomit or to eliminate the calories with the use of laxatives. These athletes may engage in excessive exercise or fasting due to a morbid fear of gaining weight. Athletic performance tends to fluctuate dramatically. Suicide attempts are common with the disorder.

None of this is good news to a parent.

Amenorrhea: Eating disorders can lead to amenorrhea, meaning the loss of the menstrual period. Nonathletic girls start their periods between the ages of twelve and fifteen, and athletes start between thirteen and fifteen and a half.

Menstruation can be delayed or disrupted as part of the female triad. Poor nutrition from eating disorders and excessive exercise contribute to the periods not starting or not occurring. Amenorrhea tends to occur when body fat percentage falls below 17 or 18 percent.

The good news is that if eating disorders are addressed appropriately, periods should begin again and normalize hormonal levels.

Osteoporosis: And the final leg of the female athlete triad is the loss of bone density. Girls (and boys) build bone during their teen years and into their twenties. We all reach our peak bone density by the time we are about thirty years old.

Imagine the damage done during these critical years when bones are not being built but are breaking down because of lack of calcium and the hormone levels needed to create bone.

Decreased estrogen associated with amenorrhea, along with decreased calcium intake from eating disorders, leads to decreased mineral content in bone. This can increase the risk of stress fractures in the female athlete with the triad. More than one stress fracture in the same athlete should raise a red flag for the parents and coaching staff.

Again, once eating disorders are under control, hormone levels and body systems can get back in line, and the cascade of problems caused by the female triad can be reversed. But treatment is necessary and critical.

Symptoms of Eating Disorders

Anorexia Nervosa:

- Weight loss
- Obsession with exercise
- Withdrawal, "loner"
- Excessive concern with weight, diet, and appearance
- Overlying sense of unhappiness
- Stress fractures, shin splints, other injuries
- Avoids social eating situations (tends to eat alone)
- Complaining of always being cold

Bulimia:

- Irregular weight loss
- Variable athletic performance
- Drug abuse
- Binge eating
- Disappears after eating (to vomit)
- Multiple complaints such as weakness, aches, and pains
- Use of laxatives

Treatment of Eating Disorders

If an athlete is suspected of having the female triad, parents, coaches, friends, and doctors are needed to help with treatment. Treatment includes a nutritional plan, emotional support, and psychiatric guidance. Hormone therapy may be necessary.

Turn first to your family doctor for a referral to an eating disorders specialist (usually you can find these mental health professionals at a major medical center or hospital system). You do not want to be referred to a dietitian or "nutritionist" because eating disorders are not about food choices.

If you are struggling with the extremes of disordered eating such as anorexia or bulimia, or if you are a concerned parent, coach, or friend, you can also turn to many national organizations for help and local referrals to specialists. These organizations are listed in the Resources section at the back of this book.

Menstrual Disorders

Problems with menstruation include both no menstruation (amenorrhea) and irregular menstruation. Amenorrhea can be primary (failure of menstruation to begin) and secondary (cessation of cycle in a girl who previously had a normal cycle). Secondary amenorrhea is defined as going three to six months or more without a menstrual cycle.

No periods or irregular periods can occur in up to 66 percent of female athletes. Compare that to only 2 to 5 percent of women in the general population. So the occurrence of menstrual problems in female athletes is quite high.

Again, girls who compete in appearance sports such as gymnastics, figure skating, dance, and endurance sports such as distance running seem to be at higher risk for menstrual problems. A girl with menstrual dysfunction is at risk for infertility, an increased incidence for heart disease, and loss of calcium in the bone. These problems are usually all reversible with the correction of the menstrual problem. However, bone mineral loss in an amenorrhea athlete can be rapid and not entirely reversible. An athlete with bone mineral loss is at higher risk for both stress fracture and fractures after trauma.

If a girl's menstrual cycle is absent for three or more months, or irregular periods are taking place, the female athlete should see a doctor. A thorough history, physical examination, and lab testing should be carried out. Depending on the specific diagnosis, treatment can include birth control pills, proper diet, and calcium supplementation. The training program needs to be addressed and decreased in some cases.

NUTRITION AND THE FEMALE ATHLETE

Male and female athletes have similar nutritional needs with the exception of iron and calcium. In female athletes with normal menstruation and estrogen levels, 1,300 mg/day of calcium is recommended. Girls with amenorrhea require 1,500 mg/day of calcium that comes from a good diet (with dairy products), which is preferred to taking calcium supplements.

Iron deficiency is found in 20 to 30 percent of female athletes. Iron can be lost through menstruation, iron-poor diet, blood loss for the gut (distance runners), sweat, and urine. High-risk athletes are endurance athletes. If a girl shows eating disorders, restrictive diet, increased fatigue, and/or decreased performance, she should be evaluated for iron deficiency anemia.

Blood tests will most likely be ordered. Iron deficiency anemia is treated with up to six months of oral iron supplements and proper diet. Iron deficiency without anemia is usually only treated with diet. Iron deficiency can usually be prevented with the proper diet.

MY MEDICAL ADVICE

A broken bone is a broken bone, whether the athlete is a boy or a girl. But sometimes girls just are different.

I see eating disorders in male athletes, especially among wrestlers and gymnasts, but eating disorders such as anorexia are much more common in females. This disorder presents a potentially life-threatening situation and should not be taken lightly.

The problem often gets ignored because the girls with this disorder are usually high achievers. They are performing well in school and sports. They also tend to be perfectionists—not an uncommon trait in athletes. They may also be obsessive about things such as washing their hands and anxious about their skin condition.

The female triad is very much tied into the diet (not eating or eating and purging), which can lead to osteoporosis and cessation of menstruation. The girls with this problem often use food and diet as a way to control this aspect of their lives when there is stress in other areas.

The exact cause of anorexia is not known, but there are often combinations of personality traits, thought processes, and environmental and physiological factors that contribute.

Parents should look for some of these symptoms and behaviors: frequent illness; unrealistic assessment of own weight; a girl who says she "feels fat"; a girl who is very fearful of gaining weight; continued diet even when a girl has lost weight; rapid weight loss; depression; obsessions; anxiety; irritability; self-esteem tied in with weight; strange eating habits (such as only eating the crust of the bread); wearing loose clothing (the sweatshirt that never comes off); feeling cold; social withdrawal; laxative or diet pill or diuretic use; perfectionism; and physical signs such as brittle hair and nails, tooth decay, swollen joints, constipation, and dry skin.

Other symptoms are confusing because they are common in all kids going through puberty and the teenage years. But these are the big behaviors to watch for. Even just a few of them would be cause to see your primary care doctor without delay.

Athletes also tend to have many of these traits such as perfectionism because they are disciplined and very competitive. Athletes who are in sports where speed is a factor are at risk. These are girls in running, swimming, and rowing. Athletes where the body form is evaluated such as gymnastics, diving, figure skating, horse riding, and dance are at risk. Both boys and girls are at risk, but girls are much more at risk, and that is why this special chapter has been devoted to them.

Extreme dieting is a much bigger risk for the female athlete, as there is also the stress of training that is placed on her body. The very process of extreme diets can lead to excessive training and poor performance. The athlete will become weak, have poor recovery, increased injury risk, and even heart irregularities. The poor nutrition and deficiency of fluid and electrolyte balance will lead to injury, fracture, illness, dehydration, and even death in some cases.

Exercise can slow down the bone loss but does not stop the process in the girl with an extreme starvation diet. Finding the girl with the eating disorder is hard to do. The diet is often a secret, and the girls, when challenged about what they are eating or not eating, state they are just "in training."

We need to instruct coaches, trainers, teammates, and family of the signs of the female triad. If your daughter is complaining about the cold, eating alone, drinking tons of water (or diet drink), using laxatives, is obsessed with diet and cooking and talking about fat all the time, please take notice. This is a serious problem, and you can save her life.

5

Would I Let My Son Play Football?

Americans love football! There is a great deal of passion surrounding the sport of football for the players and the fans. I believe that the football experience should not be taken away from the kids who want to play.

There are other, more dangerous things that your child could be doing such as riding a bike, riding a motorcycle, driving a car, or perhaps playing girls soccer (more on that later). When it comes right down to dangerous activity, there is a much greater risk of getting in a car accident on the way to the football game than your child having a significant injury in the game.

And yet …

I am often asked if I would let my son play football. The topic comes up every summer before "two-a-day" practice. The number of times that I get asked this question has increased as the concerns about concussion in football players has become a growing area of concern.

I cringe when I hear the sound of two helmets crashing together during a game or when a player goes down and takes more than two seconds to get up. When a player uses his helmet as a battering ram, I visualize the blocker's brain crashing into his skull.

I know that with every concussion there is an internal chemical reaction and cascade of symptoms that develops over time. The injury evolves over days, weeks, and possibly longer. The chemical cascade in the brain will result in cell death and diminished ability to make decisions, feel, move, balance, and remember. The player's emotions can become unpredictable.

The brain cells and connections that are lost after a concussion never regrow. We have no medications to make the injured player grow new brain cells. Thankfully, about 80 percent of players with concussion are better after about eight to ten days of rest. But there is no denying that there is a price to pay for playing an aggressive contact sport such as football.

Football has always been an aggressive collision sport. This is part of the allure of the sport to fans and participants. The sport has inherent risks for concussions and traumatic events. The repetitive hitting of the head that takes place with almost every tackle and block can result in subconcussive events. A subconcussive event is micro head trauma that occurs thousands of times during a high school or college football career.

No type of helmet or headgear can protect against this head trauma. The subconcussive events are more common than the concussions and often cause no symptoms *at the time*. However, repetitive head collisions may be the main culprit in the mental and cognitive loss and the dementia and the chronic traumatic encephalopathy (CTE) that plagues veteran football players. I'll explain CTE in a minute.

The CDC has studied more than three thousand football players. Sadly, these players die of degenerative neurological diseases such as Alzheimer's and Lou Gehrig's disease at a rate three to four times more than the general population (CDC, "NIOSH FACTS").

Boston University (BU) researchers have studied brains donated with much generosity and concern from athletes and veteran players of football (Daneshvar et al. 2011). BU reports that of the thirty-five brains donated by professional football players, thirty-four of them showed some evidence of CTE—chronic traumatic encephalopathy.

CTE is a brain disorder that is associated with the buildup of abnormal proteins called tau. Tau builds up in areas of the brain that are important for memory, decision making, and emotion. The buildup of this protein can be associated with poor concentration and headaches and later to aggressive behavior and depression.

Most of the brains in the study were from older, veteran players, but one brain was from an eighteen-year-old player. The diagnosis of CTE has been made in several former NFL players who committed suicide, including Dave Duerson, Terry Long, Andre Waters, and, more recently, Junior Seau.

The death at age forty-three of Seau, a star linebacker in the NFL, has provided insight into the long-term consequences of playing football. Although he never had a documented "concussion" with the league, it may have been just the day-to-day jarring of the head that led to brain trauma.

RISKIER ACTIVITIES (COMPARED TO FOOTBALL)

So is there a risk in playing football? Yes. Every year football players in the United States die from head trauma or sudden cardiac death or heat illness. What are the true risks of football? Head trauma is more common in bicycling than it is in football. Playground accidents are close to football in the incidence of head trauma.

Concussions may have a higher incidence in girls' soccer than in football. I can't cite any studies to support the observation about girls' soccer, but as a team doc standing on the sidelines and from talks with coaches and trainers, we see girls being injured (a higher incidence with less severity) because they literally use their heads for the sport and do not wear helmets.

You've heard some people claim that football is far too violent and should be banned as a sport. Others believe there is no other game quite like football for its outstanding benefits to players. The advocates think the risks of injuries are overblown scare tactics and should be put into the proper perspective with other sports such as boxing, soccer, lacrosse, and bicycling.

The *New Republic* published an interview with President Obama in which he was quoted as saying that he loved football but had worries about the long-term effects of the violence and hard hits of the game. President Obama went on to comment that he would have to "think long and hard" about allowing a son to play football.

Former NFL players such as Kurt Warner worry about letting their own kids play football. Matt Bowen, the former NFL safety, has remarked on many positive aspects to football but believes they must be balanced with the risks. He also has voiced concerns about his own boys playing football. Roger Goodell, NFL commissioner, states that he absolutely would want his son, if he had one, to play football.

On the positive side, there is no sport like football for building social skills and developing teamwork. I will say it again: There is simply no better sport for building teamwork. Football teaches kids about hard work, strategy, teamwork, social skills, and trust building. All of these qualities are important life lessons that provide kids with tools for all aspects of life.

As Alexander the Great said, "Upon the conduct of each depends the fate of all." This sums up the philosophy of football. There is a good reason that the first week in high school football practice is called hell week. Hell week is not meant to kill you, but it does make you wish you were dead (figure of speech).

Some of the guys may quit, but the real players are staying put and taking what the coaches throw at them. At all times, the players have a choice. They are taught to work as a team. Some coaches have the players run laps, and if one player comes in first, then they all run another lap. They are not allowed to let one player come in first or last. This is real teamwork.

Football is not for everyone, but the players who get through football training come out better for it.

There is also the social status on the high school campus of being a football player. Kids dream of playing college or professional football. For many kids, football is a ticket to a college education—not to mention fame and possible fortune in the NFL. Regardless, football offers an opportunity to many kids, and, for some, it's a way up in the world that otherwise would not exist.

NFL Commissioner Goodell has declined to confirm that there is a proven connection between football and medical problems in retired players. He has emphasized in recent interviews, however, that the NFL is supporting research to study the risks of the sport. In addition, the NFL has changed some rules to make the game safer. All this at the same time thousands of former players have filed suit against the NFL—claiming that not enough was done to inform them about the dangers of concussions and that more needs to be done now to take care of their medical needs.

To make matters worse, there is no firm evidence that protective gear, such as face guards and helmets, prevents concussions. More likely the helmet and face guard prevent external injuries to the face and head but not to the brain.

The use of protective gear, such as a helmet, may even change behavior so that the player is more aggressive—for example, when a player uses his helmet as a battering ram against the opposing player. This is a dangerous technique and puts both players at more risk. Without the helmet or face guard, a safer form of attack might be played.

TOO DANGEROUS? TOO DIRTY?

Former NCAA coach Lou Holtz stated in an interview in the *Wall Street Journal* (Moore 2013) that he is troubled by the increase in the incidence of concussions and spinal injuries in what seems to be an increasingly violent sport. Holtz also regrets that dangerous and dirty hits are often glorified on TV replays.

Coach Holtz recommends taking the "face guards off the helmets." He says, "That way players can't lunge headfirst and use the helmet as a battering ram." He also thinks that a softer helmet would lead to less violence in the game: "Players would go back to the fundamentals of tackling—no more concussions."

This is an interesting comment and has truth to it. But players are not going to take off the face guard and risk losing an eye.

The majority of people are in the middle of the debate about football. I can see the argument from many sides. Let's start with the medical side of the problem.

I am an orthopedic surgeon who takes care of injured athletes. I see patients with fractures, sprains and strains, overuse injuries, head injuries, concussions, trauma, bumps, and bruises. Some injuries are devastating. Some injuries are season ending, and some injuries are permanent.

Injured football players make up a big part of my practice, especially when practice starts in the summer and lasts until the end of the season in November.

Orthopedic complaints are not the only problems that can become long term. Dementia, CTE, emotional problems, chronic headaches, depression, a failure to deal with daily life, and even suicide can be the result of head trauma. These diagnoses are devastating.

If you don't let your boy play football, do you also stop him from riding his bike or skateboarding, driving in cars, playing soccer, and climbing on jungle gyms on the school playground? A parent cannot take away all risk from life.

The answer to the question, "Would you let your son play football?" really is not difficult for me. The answer is yes. I cannot eliminate all risk from life; all I can do is try to reduce the risks.

Education and awareness can help reduce the risks. Preseason screening, heat injury prevention, proper protective gear and equipment, appropriate tackling technique, concussion baseline testing (like the IMPACT and SCAT3) and injury monitoring are important steps to awareness.

As you would expect, reducing exposure will also reduce risk. Limiting full contact practices will reduce injury rates by reducing the number of hits. Rule changes will change the dynamics of play and reduce injury exposure. Hits to the head and hits on defenseless receivers should be penalized as dangerous techniques. Dangerous, unsportsmanlike conduct should be fined.

If there is an injury, parents, players, and coaches need to be instructed on the signs of concussion. They need to be taught how to identify them and report them, as I outlined in chapter 3.

THE CULTURE OF FOOTBALL

Keep in mind that football is not just a game. Football is a culture. There is bravado in football that cannot be matched in any other sport. The culture of football includes violence. The game is exciting to many because of the violence and not knowing if the quarterback will get back up and play.

If the violence disappears from football, does it become a game of pure skill? To be honest, if the violence were removed from football, it would not be as popular. Nobody would watch it!

There are really only a few skill positions in football. These are the positions that are the most responsible for preventing or creating points. The skill positions are quarterback, running back (halfback), wide receiver, cornerback, safety, and the return specialist. Players in the skill positions are usually smaller than the linemen and are typically faster and have other talents. But football is going through a period of momentous change. I think the game will be better for it.

The NFL has proposed safety changes. The owners outlawed peel-back blocks anywhere on the field. A peel-back block occurs when the player is moving toward his goal line, approaches an opponent from behind or the side, and makes contact with that player below the waist. This is the type of block that blasted apart Houston Texans linebacker Brian Cushing's left knee.

Overloading a formation while attempting to block a field goal or extra point is also banned.

A proposal to ban offensive players from using the crown of their helmets against defenders in the open field was controversial but will ban players from delivering forceful blows. It was the rule that provided the biggest step in safety, especially to prevent head injury and concussions. This may be a hard rule to enforce.

New York Giants coach Tom Coughlin commented, "It does reinforce the importance of getting out in front of this before something tragic happens," and added, "The verbiage from the medical people who spoke to us ... was not pretty [about potential injuries] in terms of some of these hits" (Corbett 2013).

IS FOOTBALL LOSING TURF?

Player safety is paramount with the rule changes in the NFL and will influence the younger players as well. It is too soon to confirm a link between parents' safety concerns and football's popularity. But some signs are in the wind. There are indications that fewer kids are putting on pads.

Football participation across all age ranges has decreased across the country, according to National Sporting Goods Association research. The number of people playing football dropped from 10.1 million in 2006 to 9 million in 2011.

The number of high school boys playing eleven-man football increased from 886,840 in 1992–1993 to 1,112,303 in 2008–2009, reports the National Federation of State High School Associations. But the number of football players has declined slightly during the two most recent years for which data were available: to 1,109,278 in 2009–2010 and 1,108,441 in 2010–2011, after sixteen years of previous growth.

The decrease in the number of high school kids participating in football does not seem to be as a result of school budget cutbacks. As a matter of fact, the number of high schools offering eleven-player football continues to increase, according to the National Federation data. The change in participation numbers in football may just reflect the normal cycle of class size and has not caused any alarm with the high school football programs. However, the numbers are worth watching over the next few years.

A better indication of what might happen at the high school level may be reflected in the Pop Warner and USA Football level, where kids can play tackle football around seven to nine years of age. My son started playing tackle football when he was nine years old. It was not my idea, but he did learn a thing or two. He learned about teamwork and how to listen to and respect his coach.

I should mention that was his first year and his last year playing football, although he was a pretty good safety. He also learned that he had much more passion for basketball.

Football has gone through many changes since 1905 when Teddy Roosevelt saved the sport from extinction. Football has seen the evolution of the forward pass, the introduction of the hard helmet, and the increased toughness of the sport. American football is an institution and culture in the United States. We have now come to another period of great change that includes putting player safety first. Injury prevention and awareness is a change that will increase the popularity of the sport, in my opinion.

I did allow my son to play football, and I would allow him again. He simply prefers basketball, and it has a whole lot less gear!

6

Training to Win: How to Stay Off the Injury List

If you get nothing else out of this chapter, I want you to know that kids' sports injuries can be prevented in the majority of cases. Some sports injuries can even be predicted.

Because more kids are participating year-round in multiple sports or specialized and participating in elite travel teams, the opportunity for injury has increased compared to a decade ago. It is up to the parent to be aware and to help prevent their kids from being placed on the injury list. The parents can start by not overscheduling, but I realize it may be too late to stop that runaway train.

To prevent injury, common sense should prevail.

Here are my top five recommendations for injury prevention:

1. Warm up. Don't let kids jump right into the game. A good warm-up includes stretching and should be done before every practice and game.
2. Wear the right equipment and make sure it fits. A kid should not be allowed on the field without the right gear. Every pad and eye protector should be in place before the coach allows the kid on the court.
3. Be serious about pitch counts and overdoing it with overhand throws and hits. Kids will keep going until they drop. It's up to the parents to do the count.

4. Be very aware that kids who play year-round sports need a break to recover from the activity. It is recommended that the kid have two days of rest every week from the sport—any sport and every sport. The developing body needs rest.
5. Even after an injury and recovery, the young athlete needs to gradually return to his or her sport. Before returning to sport, the kid needs full range of motion of the injured part, full strength when compared to the other side, and to have maintained the endurance needed to participate for a full practice. It may take a few weeks or a few months to ease back into a sport after an injury.

But keep in mind that the majority of kids' sports injuries can be prevented from happening in the first place.

MEET THE PLAYERS—SPORTS MEDICINE SPECIALISTS YOU WANT ON YOUR TEAM

Preventing injuries in our kids who play sports takes a village. Your kids will come in contact with many people who are part of the team, the organization, the school, and the training and medical personnel.

If your child becomes injured, another team of professionals may be involved in assessing and treating your child's injuries and helping during rehab and physical therapy.

I want to introduce the players on this important team because you need to know who they are and the extent of their medical training and what they can do—and what they should not do.

So who are the sports medicine specialists on your team?

Your family doctor or pediatrician. The family doctor is a medical doctor (MD) who specializes in family medicine. He or she is a general physician who can perform your child's preseason physical. This exam includes a sports physical that makes sure that the child's body can handle the sport and the training. Even if your state does not require a sports physical, it is a very good idea to get one before your student athlete starts the season.

Here's what to expect during the sports physical, also known as the preparticipation examination. The doctor evaluates the child's health and overall fitness and also how the child's condition relates to the sport. The doc will be looking to see if your child has any illness or disorder such as a heart condition that might make your child's participation in sports unsafe.

Many schools will set up the sports physical with the physician or physicians visiting the school. There may be stations set up for various tests, such as blood pressure. A physician's assistant or a nurse practitioner may help with the evaluation.

Usually the examination is done about six weeks before the season starts, and if your child has any problems that need treating, you will have time to take care of them.

The exam starts with a thorough medical history that includes a history of medical illnesses, vaccinations, hospital stays, injuries, and accidents. Often you can answer many of these questions by filling out the answers on a medical questionnaire. If this isn't your regular doctor, you'll want to get a listing of vaccinations and dates before this preseason exam and bring it along.

The illnesses and problems that are asked about include the following: shortness of breath, asthma, dizziness, fainting, diabetes, excess fatigue, frequent headaches, eating disorder, vision problems (wear glasses or contacts), epilepsy, heart problems such as murmur or irregular rhythm, past surgery, broken bones, torn ligaments and tendons, injuries, accidents, hospitalizations, concussions, joint injuries, spine injuries, back pain, skin problems, anxiety, digestion problems, severe allergies, liver or kidney problems, medications that your child takes regularly, family history of heart problems or sudden death before the age of fifty, and diet.

Your child may not know some of the answers (and the parent can prompt or respond), but for most kids, the doc wants to know the responses from the child (as hard as this may be for many parents). Also consider that the child may have different responses if the parent is present in the exam room. Respect your child's privacy—to a point.

The medical examination will include these measures: height, weight, pulse, blood pressure, heart exam, and lung exam. The doctor will perform neurologic function testing of reflexes, coordination, balance, and strength. Eyes (vision) and ears (hearing) will be checked along with a look in the ears, nose, and throat. The doctor will test the child's joint range of motion, flexibility, spinal alignment, instability of joints, posture, and gait; and some exams will include blood tests for cholesterol, hemoglobin, and anemia. The child may be asked to leave a urine specimen.

Girls will be asked about their periods as to when they started and if they are regular.

Additional tests such as an EKG (to check the heart electrically), x-rays, and more blood tests may be ordered.

A more detailed preseason physical may include sports-specific drills such as jumping height, hop test, and even SCAT3 or IMPACT tests of brain function.

The physician will then decide whether it is safe for your child to participate. The doctor may consider the type of sport, the position played, level of competition, size and maturity of the athlete, and the ability to modify the sport and wear protective gear.

If everything is fine, the preseason physical will be signed off. But recommendations may be made such as bringing an inhaler (for allergies and asthma) to a game or an epinephrine auto-injector (EpiPen) if your child reacts to insect bites.

For minor sports injuries during practice or a game, such as a sprained ankle or a cut, you can see your family doctor. If this primary care doc can't handle a certain type of injury, make sure this doctor refers you to the appropriate specialist.

The Emergency Room doctor. Let's hope you don't get to meet any of the ER docs, but if your child ends up in the Emergency Department, here's what might happen. The ER doc will triage the injury and order x-rays or an MRI or CT.

The ER doctor will order necessary tests to assess the injury and order initial treatment. The ER doctor will usually set up a follow-up visit and refer to a specialist if that is needed. The ER doctor's job is to make sure your child is not in a life-threatening situation. If the ER doc can patch the kid up, your injured athlete might be sent home with instructions about PRICE MM (rest, ice, and pain medications, explained in a previous chapter as the first line of care for many sports injuries and a method of home care) and sent home with the parents.

At that point, the injury becomes the problem of the child and parents and must be reported to the coaching team and a plan for return to play developed.

For serious injuries, the child might be admitted to the hospital, and a specialist, an orthopedic surgeon like myself, is called in. My partners and I respond to requests for broken bones, dislocated knees and other joints, neck and back injuries, any fracture that has bone sticking out of the skin (called an open fracture), and any fracture that is associated with severe swelling or nerve damage. A neurosurgeon may be called in to examine the player and the MRI or CT scan if there is suspected brain or spinal cord injury, for example.

The specialist. A medical specialist is a doctor who has completed advanced extra education and clinical training in a specific area of medicine (their specialty). There are many examples of medical specialists including the orthopedic surgeon, hand surgeon, dentist, internist, cardiologist, neurosurgeon, and pediatrician.

If you are working with a specialist, that doctor will follow your child through the injury. For a broken leg, for example, the specialist might perform surgery or set the broken leg in a cast. You will see this doctor several times to monitor the healing of the bone or growth plate injury.

At some point our job as specialists is finished. We might advise what type of rehabilitation program your child should be doing, and we would refer you to the appropriate rehab and physical therapy clinics.

The team doctor. The team doctor is the doctor for a sports team who is in charge of medical services and coverage for a sports team. He or she will often sit on the bench with the team and respond to an injured player during a game. For high school and club teams, most of these doctors are volunteers.

As a team doctor, I'm on the sidelines during the games and sometimes during practice. I monitor any injured players to make sure they have completed any rehab from an injury. During a game I can respond to an injury on the field. I can evaluate the player after he or she comes off the field. It is not unusual to suture a player in the training room, if the kid has sustained a laceration during play.

Your team doctor may work closely with the team trainer. They will consult each other about injured players and return to play schedules and will put together a good strength and conditioning program for the team. This is important for prevention and overall health of the players. The team physician may have examined every player during the preseason physicals.

Emergency Medical Technician (EMT). These are the people who come with the ambulance and provide urgent medical care to injured players, or they are privately hired medical people who work the sidelines during a game. The EMT is usually very physically fit, as they are often required to lift and carry people. Many high schools have EMTs providing medical coverage at football games. The EMT on the sidelines can call an ambulance, if necessary. It is not unusual to have an ambulance on the sidelines for a game as well.

The EMTs have the training and the equipment to take care of catastrophic and noncatastrophic injuries. It is up to the home team to hire emergency personnel and for the school board, in many cases, to vote on the guidelines for having EMTs present during games.

Physical therapists (PT). These medical personnel help players who have been injured improve their motion and manage pain. They play an important part in rehabilitation and return to the game. Physical therapists usually work in a private office or clinic and spend most of their time actively working with patients. The PT will help with specific exercises, manual therapy, and manipulation and will use tools such as ultrasound to decrease pain and swelling.

PTs are an important part of rehabilitation after an injury. Typically your child may visit them two to three times a week for about four to six weeks after a serious orthopedic injury, for example.

Coach. The team coach will help the players work toward building their full potential and work as a member of a team. The coach will help each player build physical and mental fitness.

The coach has an ethical and legal obligation to the players. Many coaches are volunteers and work other paid jobs. Many coaches work part time. They develop and teach the understanding of fitness, injury, mental toughness, nutrition, and sports science. The coach should be able to evaluate performance and provide appropriate feedback and balance criticism with positive comments to motivate the team.

The coach should be a good communicator so that his or her instructions are understood. Coaches should be able to demonstrate the sport or routine by breaking it down into sequence like a science. Encouragement of players' goals is important. A good coach knows the sport and the rules of the game and many have been former players. A good coach is a motivator and can make practice challenging and fun. A good coach can listen and motivate. Great coaches are role models and are remembered fondly by the players.

Team trainers. The team trainer will deliver emergency care, develop injury prevention programs, and provide some prevention services such as tape. Trainers will help with rehabilitation of the injured athlete under the direction of a licensed physician.

The team trainer is an ATC (certified athletic trainer) and will put together the fitness program for many high school teams. The trainer provides athletic training for all home games and away varsity games. The team trainer acts as a link among the physician and the team, the parents, and other medical specialists.

Certified athletic trainers are highly educated and skilled professionals who specialize in athletic health care. The athletic trainer is the person responsible for the players' health care, from injury prevention programs to injury rehabilitation programs, first aid, injury management, and evaluation of players' injuries, especially if there is no team doctor.

The National Athletic Trainers Association (NATA) requires that certified athletic trainers take written and oral examinations to test their skills in the following five areas:

1. Prevention
2. Recognition, evaluation, and immediate care of athletic injuries
3. Rehabilitation and reconditioning of athletic injuries
4. Health care delivery
5. Education and development of athletic program

Most often, trainers will maintain an accurate list of injuries and treatments.

Registered Dietitian. A lot of people think they know a lot about nutrition and food choices. Millions of books and diet plans profess to have "the answer." The only qualified people to offer nutritional advice are registered dietitians (experts with RD credentials).

The people at the nutrition and health food store or the supplement/nutrition store, the whole foods devotees, and the "nutritionist" are not generally experts. They will load you up with supplements and protein concoctions your players don't know, need, or understand.

There is a difference between a registered dietitian and someone who calls himself or herself a nutritionist. It's depth of training and knowledge. Rely on experts. These days you can tap into the expertise of an RD at your grocery store or through your child's doctor's office. Many hospital systems have RDs on staff for you, as do children's hospitals. Ask your family doctor for a referral if you have nutritional questions and concerns.

Girls (and sometimes boys) with suspected eating disorders such as anorexia or bulimia need to be seen by a psychologist first. These are often psychological issues that will eventually need a team of mental health experts and dietitians. Certain sports are known to foster eating and weight loss issues (gymnastics, diving, running, wrestling, cheerleading, and figure skating).

The triad of eating disorders is discussed in much more depth in the chapter on female athletes, and I urge you to take action if you suspect your child (usually a daughter) might have these concerns.

Parents. Whether you think so or not, you as a parent are a vital member of your child's sports team. You get up early to drive the kids to practice. You sit long hours on the sidelines during practice and games. You're the head cheerleader. You bring treats to the team. You write checks for equipment and fees.

And when it comes to prevention, no one is going to worry about your child getting injured on that field more than you are. As chief worrier, you are the one to remind your child to drink water, to clean his or her equipment, to check that shoes are fitting properly or buy new ones, to serve healthy foods when it's so much easier to drive through and dine on the dashboard.

Don't underestimate your role in helping prevent injuries.

First responders. Whether it's a team doctor on the sidelines, a trainer, or a trained professional medical first responder in the stands, someone must know how to perform CPR and use an AED (automated external defibrillator). Most schools have AEDs, and all athletic venues need to have one available. You don't want to wait for the ambulance paramedics or EMTs or police car to arrive with an AED when precious minutes tick by without one.

A fully stocked first aid kit is an essential too. It's a fair question at a parent meeting to ask about safety precautions, including the availability of a first aid kit and AED. Expect a complete answer, and don't let the coaching staff get away with, "Oh, yah, we have that."

Coaches and trainers and the team doctor should have this vital medical information at all practices and games:

- Medical history cards: An alphabetical card file box should be available to each coach, trainer, and athletic director with medical information for each athlete.
- Informed parental consent and acknowledgment of risk forms signed by the athletes and parent/guardian
- Insurance information for all athletes on file
- Physical forms on file
- Injury report forms for record keeping
- Athletes with special needs should have a form that needs to be flagged, and coaching staff and trainers must be aware of athletes participating in sports with special medical needs such as asthma, epilepsy, and diabetes. There should be a "quick reference" for all special needs players that is easy to find.
- Emergency action plan for home and away games. This plan must be in writing so that there is no confusion during an emergency. Staff in service and the plan should be in writing for all coaches and administrators.
- CPR and first aid certificates for all coaches

The first aid kit on the field should include the following supplies, all updated, fresh, clean, and with personnel trained to administer first aid:

Safety pins
EMT scissors/shears
First Aid Manual and CPR Flash Cards
Sharp-pointed surgical scissors
Bandage scissors
Splinter forceps
Oral thermometer (also surface thermometers)
Tongue depressors

Flashlight that is waterproof or a headlight
CPR mouth barrier
Sterile gloves, at least two pairs
Instant cold packs/chemical type
Plastic bags for ice
Rescue blanket
Cell phone
Medical release forms
List of emergency phone numbers for paramedics, hospital ER, police, poison control
Elastic bandages of various sizes including 4-inch and 6-inch
Adhesive strips for wound closure of various sizes and skin glue
4 x 4 and 5 x 9 and 8 x 10 gauze, four packets minimum of each
Sterile gauze rolls of various sizes 1, 2, 3, and 4 inches
Nonstick sterile bandages, Telfa of various sizes
1-inch rolled cloth adhesive tape
1-inch rolled paper or silk (hypoallergenic) tape
1-inch rolled waterproof tape
1-inch rolled conforming gauze, known as C-tape
Molefoam ($4\frac{1}{8}$-inch x $3\frac{3}{8}$-inch size)
Moleskin Plus ($4\frac{1}{8}$-inch x $3\frac{3}{8}$-inch size)
Spenco 2nd skin and Spenco Adhesive knit bandages
Tegaderm transparent wound dressing
Liquid soap and hand sterilizer
Sterile disposable surgical brush
Sterile cotton tipped swabs, 2 per package
Tincture of benzoin, bottle or swab sticks
Providien iodine 10 percent solution, 1 oz. bottle or swab sticks
Antiseptic towelettes
Tourniquet
Cravat cloth (triangle bandages)
Elastic wrap, Ace type in 2-, 3- and 4-inch wrap
SAM splints in 4-inch x 36-inch size (2)
Aluminum finger splints
Sterile prepackaged oval eye pads

Eye bandages, prepackages, Coverlet eye Occlusor
Metal or plastic eye shield
Sterile eyewash, 1 oz.
Contact lens remover
Bacitracin, bacitracin-neomycin polymyxin B sulfate ointment
Insect repellant with DEET
Sunscreen lotion or cream (SF 15 or 30)
Lip balm or sunscreen
Sunblock
Ibuprofen 200 mg tablets
Acetaminophen 325 mg tablets
Antacid
Decongestant (such as oxymetazoline) nasal spray (to treat nose bleed that doesn't respond to simple pressure)
Glucose (liquid glucose) paste tube to treat hypoglycemia, low blood sugar
Metered dose to bronchodilator (albuterol) to treat asthma attack
Peak flow meter
EpiPen Auto-Injector (0.3 mg) and EpiPen Jr., Auto-Injector (0.15 mg), or allergy kit with injectable epinephrine (AnaKit)
Diphenhydramine (Benadryl) 25 mg capsules

If you don't see a well-stocked kit like this on the sidelines, it's a fair question to ask the coaches why not. And if you really want to force the issue, which I think is worth forcing, show them the list in this book.

Now that you've met the real "team," I want to discuss the areas of prevention of injury. You'll see these players popping up in this discussion because they all have continuing roles to play.

But let us not minimize the role of the young athletes themselves. They are out there kicking and hitting and running and throwing. Sometimes they don't know the dangers inherent in their "play." That's why it's so important for them to be as fully prepared for battle on the field of play. Strength and conditioning are vital to their success—and key to injury prevention.

MUSCLE UP: A STRENGTH AND CONDITIONING GUIDE FOR YOUNG ATHLETES

Strength and conditioning programs for young athletes are being recognized as a means to prevent or reduce injuries. Studies have been published in soccer and football that demonstrate lower injury rates in teams that have a strength and conditioning program.

The first goal of strength and conditioning is certainly to reduce or prevent injuries. The second goal is to increase sports performance. Not the other way around.

Stronger neck muscles through strength training, for example, will decrease the acceleration and deceleration forces of the head and brain and may help prevent a concussion. Sports performance with conditioning can be improved with an increase in vertical jump, explosive power, and strength of muscles around the knee, shoulder, and spine—with some injury prevention built in.

A strength and conditioning program will improve the motor skills involved in the major movements of a sport. Young athletes need to learn the skills for their sport and also how to warm up, stretch, strength train, and develop power, agility, toughness, and explosiveness.

Strength training with weights and conditioning that includes stretching are key to proper development of the young athlete.

Strength/Resistance Training

Muscles get stronger and bigger if they are used. Put muscles under a little stress, and they'll grow even more. That's simply the point of strength training with weights. Lifting (or resisting) weights puts muscles under stress to cause them to grow.

Strength and resistance training can be used to enhance athletic and sports performance. It can also be used to prevent injury and for rehabilitation after an injury.

Types of Strength and Resistance Exercises

- Body weight resistance such as push-ups and pull-ups
- Free weights such as dumbbells and bars
- Weight machines in which you can adjust the weight
- Resistance bands (elastic tubing or bands like bungee cords)
- Medicine balls (heavy leather balls about the size of a basketball filled with sand, they don't bounce)
- Machines such as the Pilates reformer that require the user to resist body weight with bands and pulleys

The mechanism behind building muscle is this: When your child lifts free weights such as dumbbells or bars or does any resistance training with bands, for example, he or she is going to push the muscles to fatigue. That's the point where the kid cannot lift one more time. The muscle is then considered to be at the point of fatigue. That's where muscle growth begins.

Weight Training Terms to Know

Resistance: Resistance exercises are known as strength training and are performed to increase the strength and mass of muscles and bone strength. The exercises help the ability of muscles to generate force. Methods for resistance training include free weights, weight machines, and calisthenics.

Fatigue: Muscle fatigue is the decline in the ability of a muscle to develop force.

Rep: A rep is one complete motion of an exercise. The number of reps you should do depends on where you are in your training and what your goals are.

Set: A set is a group of consecutive repetitions (reps).

Maximum load: The maximum amount of weight that one can lift in a single repetition for a given exercise.

It is important to note that the high school athlete who does not have significant weight training or weight lifting experience should be considered a beginner. A beginner should develop technique and speed first. Absolute strength, however, will come later as the athlete matures and begins strength training.

Young athletes need to learn how to lift, just as they would have to learn any skill for their sport. It is important, however, that the competitive kid avoid pushing his or her maximum efforts too often. This applies to maximum weight and number of repetitions with a given weight.

The more fatigued the young athlete becomes in training, the longer the recovery period will be. The adolescent athlete cannot be trained as often as the adult. The volume (sets and reps) and the intensity (weight) used in strength training may be reduced by the coach or trainer to allow for quicker recovery in a young athlete.

Benefits of Resistance Training

Resistance and strength training are used to improve sports performance, recover from injury, prevent injury, gain strength, train muscles through neuromuscular education, and increase size and enhance explosiveness.

Studies have reported that resistance and strength training can be used safely in kids (Falk and Tenenbaum 1996; Fleck and Kraemer 1997; Payne et al. 1997). Any gains that have been made in a strength program need to be maintained, or those gains will be lost in about six weeks. Just as with adults, "use it or lose it" still applies.

Not that long ago—okay thirty years ago and more—it was thought that resistance training for young athletes was risky, that it would retard skeletal growth and cause injuries. School programs never included weights or resistance training. There were no machines or dumbbells. Those were only for the mysterious world of bodybuilders and pro wrestlers and big guys at Venice Beach who read *Muscle & Fitness* magazine.

Fast forward to gyms and health clubs today where men and women of all sizes and shapes and goals are clanging the bars and hitting the weight benches.

The same goes for the world of kids and weights. Research changed all that old thinking, and now kids can gain strength well before puberty with an appropriate and supervised weight training program.

Although there's no magic age when kids can start using weights with resistance, kids as young as six or seven can start. They must be able to follow direction and enjoy participation.

Just understand that their gains in strength are not from building monster-sized muscles but from neuromuscular education, which leads to an increase in the number of nerves that will fire with each muscle action. It's a way of training nerves and muscles to perform a movement, such as perfecting that fastball in pitching. Some people call this muscle memory.

Before puberty, all kids have low hormone (androgen) levels, but still gain from strength training because of the neuromuscular training. Some increase in muscle size, however small, still occurs in this young age group with strength training.

Enter hormones. Those same horrible hormones that create pimples and grumpy teens help build their muscles. Circulating testosterone is necessary to see a significant increase in muscle size. In females, natural growth hormones may help increase strength from resistance workouts.

Interestingly, the National Electronic Injury Surveillance System of the Consumer Product Safety Commission reports injury rates in kids are caused because they don't use the equipment properly and because of poor supervision. You'll want to insist that the coaching staff and trainers are on the site, spotting and guiding while the team is working out with weights.

Gym memberships for kids ages six to seventeen are on the rise. Whether your kids are training with the team or at a private club or YMCA, make sure they are shown how to use the equipment and have a workout plan. Each student athlete needs a written worksheet to track equipment, weight settings, and dates to record the number of sets and reps.

Strength training is a common part of training in football and wrestling in which size and strength are prized. Yet strength training may improve running speed, jumping skills, and performance in all sports

(Malina 2006). And as I've been stressing, strength training may help prevent sports injury as well.

The use of anabolic steroids and other body-building supplements such as testosterone should be discussed with your kids. If a young athlete wants to improve size and strength, he or she should be told about the physical, mental, and legal risks and real dangers of using performance-enhancing drugs.

Kids should begin a strength program with low-resistance exercises only when proper technique has been mastered. Weight can be increased in small increments once eight to fifteen repetitions can be performed. All muscle groups should be exercised through the full range of motion.

A workable program would last twenty to thirty minutes, two to three times a week. That's all the time commitment needed to show improvement. As strength gains are made, weight and repetitions can be added. Qualified supervision is required. Strength training more than four times per week does not offer any advantage. Muscles need a day of rest after a workout day.

One of the first papers showing the benefits of resistance training in kids was a report in the *Journal of Pediatric Orthopedics* in 1986 (Sewall and Micheli). Since then, many researchers have reported that a good strength and resistance program can improve strength in kids. An improvement in strength of approximately 30 percent is common even after a short period of strength training (lasting eight to twenty weeks).

But note, if training stops, preadolescents lose strength gains faster than adolescents. The most important message is that kids need to be supervised with any strength training program.

Sports performance in the young athlete comes from practice and perfecting the skills of the specific sport more than from strength training. However, strength training, sport-specific skills practice, and a sound aerobic program is the best combination for any athlete to improve his or her performance.

Benefits of Resistance Training for Young Athletes

- Improves muscle power and coordination
- Improves heart health along with aerobic exercise
- Helps prevent sports injuries by strengthening vulnerable body parts, hardens them for impact and overuse
- Strengthens bones through impact on the frame that stimulates bone growth
- May increase insulin sensitivity (avoid diabetes) and decrease body fat
- An added benefit for obese kids because of the insulin sensitivity reduction; makes more sense for obese kids who have difficulty running to stick with strength training
- Can protect the ACL (anterior cruciate ligament in the knee) when combined with plyometrics, especially in female athletes
- Improves bone mineral content of developing bones when combined with aerobic exercise

What are the risks with resistance training?

Dropping a dumbbell on a toe is a real risk. But the benefits of strength training far outweigh any risks—even a bruised toe.

The National Strength and Conditioning Association and the American Academy of Pediatrics have reported some potential problems with adolescent weight training. Lack of supervision and minimal instruction may be the biggest problems (Faigenbaum et al. 2009).

You know how it goes in the gym: Kids become competitive with each other and may push up the weight. Kids may horse around in the weight room. These behaviors can lead to injury. The immature athlete should be trained in a safe environment. Maximum lifts should not be required until the athlete is mature.

A free-weight program is considered by most strength coaches to be the most effective way to train a young athlete. Machines do not always have a carry-over effect to sports performance. Machines do not always fit the body of the immature athlete because weight machines are often designed for adult bodies. Machines may provide only one exercise per machine.

Gyms and health clubs that cater to women (smaller women) may have smaller machines better suited to teen-sized bodies.

Case reports are rarely reported on weight lifting injuries in kids of all ages. Injuries to the growth plate in the wrist make up most of these reports. These injuries were mostly preventable by avoiding maximum lifts, practicing good technique, and having appropriate supervision.

One study looked at youth sports injuries over a one-year period and found only 0.7 percent of 1,576 injuries (that's just eleven kids) related to resistance training (Malina 2006). In the same study, football accounted for 19 percent of injuries, basketball 15 percent, and soccer 2 percent. Significantly higher rates of injury are seen in kids using exercise equipment at home.

There has been no scientific proof that weight lifting or resistance training is harmful to growth or cardiovascular health in kids. All kids, however, should be cleared by a doctor before participation in a sports training program, and weight lifting is no exception.

Overuse injuries can occur with strength training, but most are related to poor training technique and supervision. Low back pain and shoulder pain are the most common areas of overuse for strength and conditioning exercises.

Trainers and coaches will understand the best techniques. For example, during the bench press, weights should always be handed off to the trainer or experienced training partner. The young athlete should primarily use a flat bench while performing the bench press (Fees et al. 1998).

Weight Lifting Checklist for Kids

With good technique and appropriate precautions, including supervision by coaches and trainers or parents, strength training programs are safe and helpful for kids in sports with these precautions:

- Kids need a preseason sports physical to be cleared to play (and train).
- Avoid power lifting, bodybuilding, and maximal lifts until growth is complete.

- Football is not the only sport that benefits from strength training. Athletes in all sports need to be strong and in great condition to play their best.
- Strength and resistance programs should include a warm-up (at least five to ten minutes) and cool-down period with less intense exercises such as light aerobics and static stretching (stretch and hold but not bouncing) while muscles are still warm.
- A proper strength and resistance program should include all important muscle groups and work through a complete range of motion.
- Any soreness, pain, or injury should be reported to the trainer, coach, parent, or facility supervisor.
- Student athletes need to focus on technique not weight. Start with light loads. Try one to three sets of six to fifteen reps of each exercise. Increase resistance gradually (only 5 to 10 percent maximum increase at one time).
- Use good muscle balance and develop core strength first.
- Strength train two or three times a week with rest days in between.
- Monitor progress with individual logs for date, sets, reps, and weight on which machines or muscle groups.
- Drink water before, during, and after the workout.

Source: Committee on Sports Medicine and Fitness, 2000–2001.

CONDITIONING FOR THE YOUNG ATHLETE

The majority of kids will have a good time playing sports, especially when they prepare for the activity. Kids should acquire skills, train their bodies, and learn to protect themselves so they are less at risk for injury. This is important for every sport, not just contact sports such as football and wrestling or highly technical sports such as gymnastics.

Young athletes need to learn the skills for their sport and also how to warm up, stretch, strength train, and develop power, agility, toughness, and explosiveness. Weight lifting (as discussed in the previous section), conditioning, and stretching are keys to proper development of the young athlete.

Unlike strength training and weight lifting, conditioning is all about body movements that increase athletic skill and physical fitness and decrease the chance of injury. The types of conditioning exercises may be different depending on the fitness goals.

To improve athletic performance, the athlete uses targeted, specific movement to mimic the moves used on the court or field. A basketball player can practice shooting baskets repeatedly to help with sports conditioning. However, aerobic conditioning—an important part of any general conditioning program—increases cardiovascular endurance and lung capacity. Usually the aerobic conditioning includes low-intensity, long-duration exercises such as running or cycling. The heart rate should be increased and sustained for a time period that challenges the heart and lungs so they get stronger.

There is also anaerobic conditioning for sports that require intense, sudden bursts of speed and strength. Weight training and sprinting are anaerobic exercises. One of the main goals of a conditioning program is to increase the amount of stress that the body can handle before it gets injured. Therefore, conditioning programs play an important role in preventing injury.

Warm-Ups (But Not Stretching)

A proper warm-up for sports should increase the blood flow to the working muscles, which will in turn lead to a decrease in muscle stiffness and less risk of injury. The warm-up will also improve performance and add to the athletes' preparation mentally before practice or a game.

The muscle temperature will rise, and, therefore, speed and strength are improved. Muscle elasticity is improved with the increase in body temperature. The blood vessels dilate, and resistance to blood flow decreases.

A good way to warm up cold muscles and get the circulation going is about ten minutes of light running (a slow jog) or cycling before practice. For runners, a jog and a few sprints thrown in is a good warm-up. It is a good idea to do gradual aerobic exercise to warm up before stretching, as the muscles will be warmed up and respond better. Jumping rope is a good substitute for running, and a jump rope is easy to stow in a sports bag if the kids' team or school doesn't have equipment.

Stretching can be used as a warm-up as well but is more effective for flexibility when done *after* a practice or workout. According to many studies, an active warm-up is more helpful than static stretching to prevent injury and soreness.

A warm-up is more important than stretching before an event. The most important benefit from stretching is obtained after the sport is played. Stretching "cold" muscles/soft tissues can lead to injury. Save the stretching for the cool-down period.

Routine stretching and stretching after a practice or game will improve flexibility. Improved flexibility may help prevent injury. The ideal time to stretch for increased flexibility is after a workout. All major muscle groups should be stretched slowly and carefully. The trainers should show proper technique, and that means the kids should not bounce while stretching. Each stretch should be held for about twenty to thirty seconds.

In general, be sure to warm up before doing any stretches. A good warm-up is slowly running in place, walking briskly, or riding a stationary bike for five to ten minutes. Speed is not important. Never bounce on a stretch because it can cause muscle strains and other injuries. After an injury, stretching may aggravate an existing injury and should not be started until advised by your doctor.

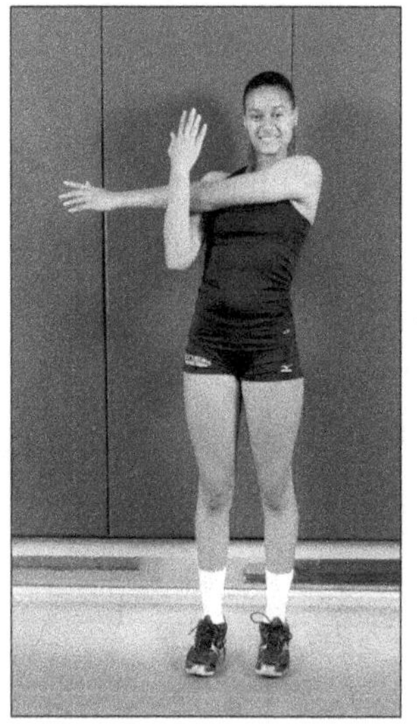

Shoulder stretch: This stretches the back of your shoulder. In a standing position, bring the first arm across your chest while using your second arm to pull it toward your chest. You will feel the stretch in the back of your shoulder. After fifteen to thirty seconds of stretching your first shoulder, switch arms.

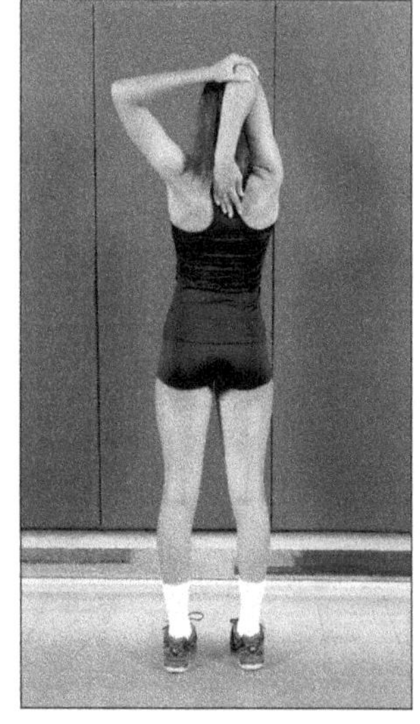

Triceps stretch: This is done in the standing position. Bring your first arm up and place the palm of your hand down the center of the back with the elbow in the air. Place your other hand on your elbow and gently hold in place as you stretch your triceps. After fifteen to thirty seconds, switch arms.

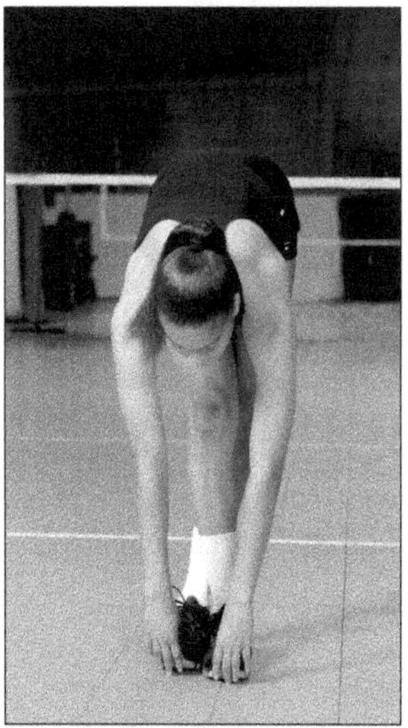

Crossover: Stand with the legs crossed and keep the feet close together and the legs straight. Try to touch your toes. Hold for five seconds and repeat three to five times and then repeat on the opposite leg.

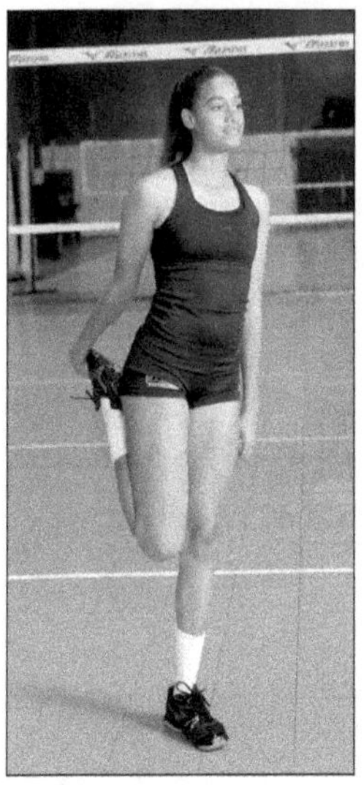

Standing quad stretch: Stand with support by holding onto a wall or a chair, if you need to. Pull the foot behind you to the buttock. Try to keep the knees close together. Hold this position for five seconds and repeat three to five times.

Forward lunges: Kneel on the right leg and place the left leg forward at a right angle. Lunge forward and keep the back leg straight. The stretch should be felt in the right groin. Hold for five seconds. Repeat three to five times and then switch legs.

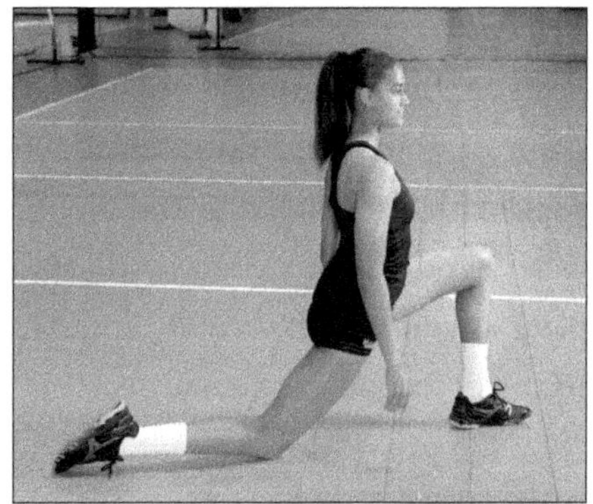

Sitting side straddle: Sit on the floor with the legs wide apart and spread. Place both hands on the same shin or ankle. Bring the chin toward the knee and keep the leg straight. Hold for five seconds and repeat three to five times. Repeat the exercise on the opposite leg.

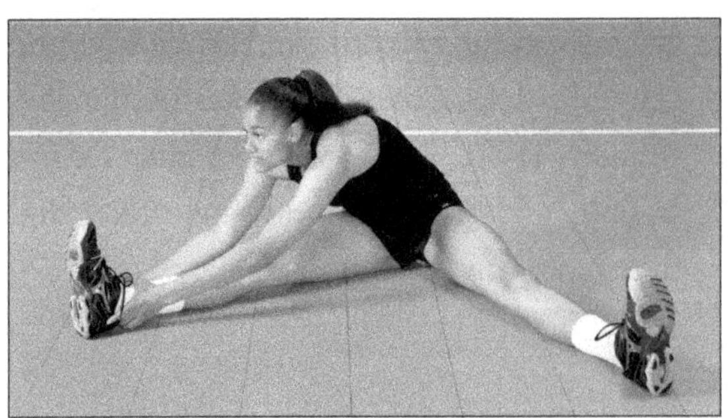

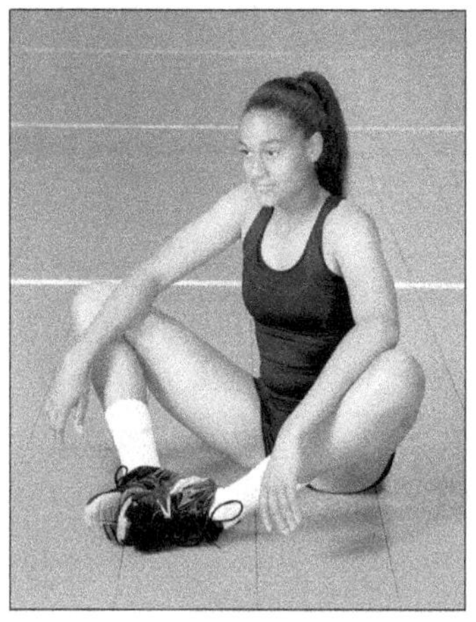

Sitting straddle butterfly: Sit on the floor with the soles of the feet touching and drop the knees toward the floor. Place the forearms on the inside of the knees and push the knees toward the ground and then lean forward from the hips. Hold for five seconds and repeat three to five times.

Sitting stretch: Sit on the floor with the legs together, feet flexed, and the hands on the shins or the ankles. Bring the chin toward the knees. Hold for five seconds and repeat three to five times.

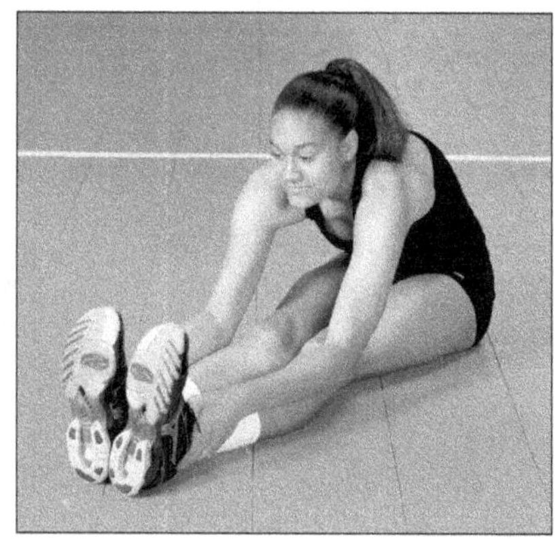

Piriformis and gluteal stretch: Lie on your back and cross the right ankle over the left knee. Grip the thigh of your left leg and pull the knee toward you, lifting the foot off the floor. Pull the knee further toward your chest to increase the stretch. Hold for between ten and thirty seconds and switch legs.

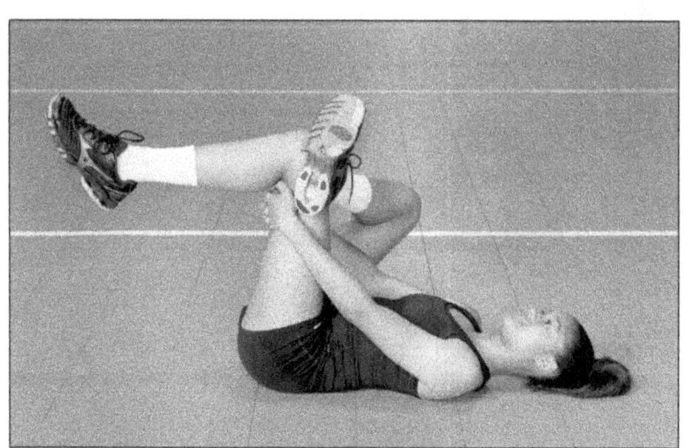

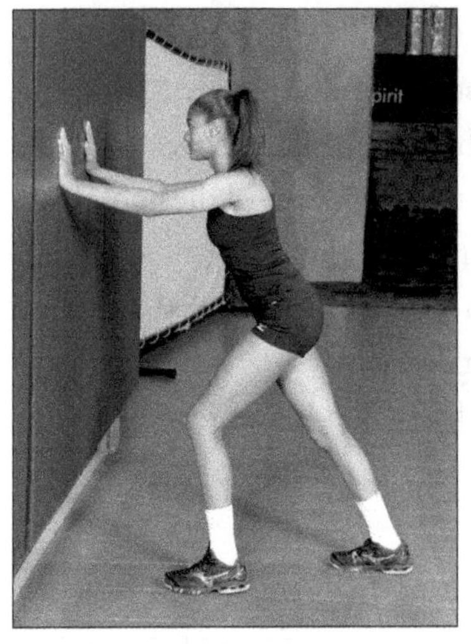

Calf stretch: Stand facing a wall with your hands on the wall at about eye level. Put the leg you want to stretch about a step behind your other leg. Keep the heel on the back leg on the floor, bend your front knee until you feel a stretch in the back leg. Hold the stretch for fifteen to thirty seconds and repeat.

Illiotibial (IT) band stretch with foam roller: Roll your leg over the foam roller (A and B), to help mobilize your tissues and break up scar tissue. Start with a sixty-second roll on each side.

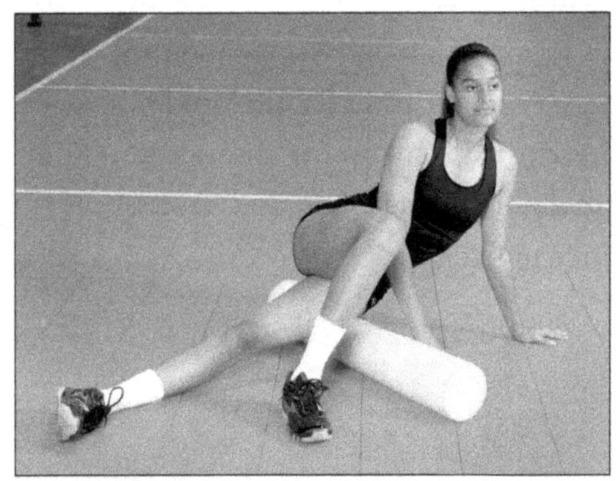

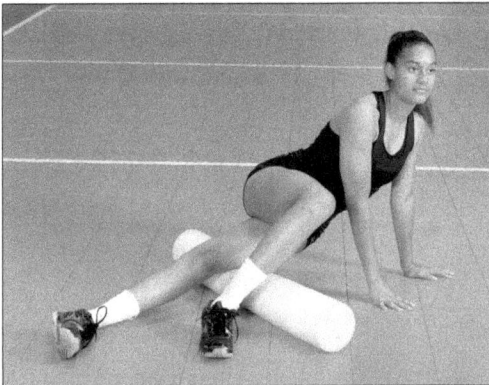

A

B

Agility and Speed Training

Agility and speed training is probably the most important training that any athlete, except swimmers, will benefit from. (Swimmers are already doing a non-land-based form of aerobic conditioning.) This should be done during the season and off-season. If the child has an opportunity to play another sport, it is suggested that he or she sign up for track and field (unless that is their primary sport, of course) because this activity provides excellent aerobic conditioning.

Studies on adult athletes have noted that if performance is the goal, cross-training may not be that helpful. No matter what the age, endurance athletes may not be helped by an alternate sport (Kolata 2011). However, one study found that resistance training improved endurance in running and cycling (Tanaka et al. 1993). Squats with heavy weights improved running.

Again, this does not work for swimmers, however; they get faster only when they do resistance training in the water that puts focus on the movements that are used in the stroke. Runners can augment their leg muscles with the muscularity they get with resistance work. But with swimmers, the research notes that mastery of the technical swimming stroke is the most important factor in performance and endurance.

Ultimately, cross-training may decrease the risk of injury in every age group simply because the primary sport is being played less.

Plyometric Exercises

Is *plyometrics* a new word for you? Quite simply, plyometric describes an explosive jump.

Many sports programs use plyometric exercises to build power, explosiveness, speed, strength, agility, and coordination. Plyometric exercises develop the high-intensity, explosive contractions of the muscles and the reflex for stretch. Stretching of the muscle before it contracts allows it to use greater force to contract. This is called the stretch reflex.

So what might this look like in action?

Plyometric exercises are usually started in high school sports and include hops, jumps, and bounding movements. A common plyometric exercise might be jumping off a box onto the floor and then rebounding onto a higher box.

These are effective exercises to improve strength, explosiveness, and sports performance. It must be pointed out that plyometric exercises are tough training techniques (they generate great force in the gluteals, hamstrings, and quadriceps) and if done incorrectly or performed without experienced supervision can be risky. Plyometric exercises are recommended for the well-conditioned kid who is involved in a sport that requires jumping and landing such as volleyball and basketball.

Plyometric exercises can be fun, safe, and helpful for young athletes when the exercise is appropriately supervised and designed (Hertling and Kessler 1996). The most important thing for coaches and trainers to teach is the proper landing technique.

The student athlete should learn to land gently on the toes and then roll back to the heels. The whole foot is used for landing, and this larger surface area spreads the impact of the force throughout the foot and the joints of the lower extremity. It is also important to avoid twisting or any sideways motion around the knee.

The proper landing technique is especially important for girls because around puberty girls tend to land in a more knock knee position than boys, which puts more stress on the knee and the ACL (anterior cruciate ligament).

Young athletes who perform plyometric exercises need to have very strong muscles prior to doing the exercises. They should warm up and start slowly with small jumps. Allow resting periods between plyometric workouts. The exercises should be performed only on a cushioned mat with well-cushioned and stable shoes.

Plyometrics are dynamic exercises with rapid eccentric and concentric muscle action. These two terms—*eccentric* and *concentric*—describe the action of the muscle. Rapid muscle movement in, say, a squat jump shows how high forces are generated in the muscle tissue. Building this movement helps with coordination during sports and mimics the types of movements

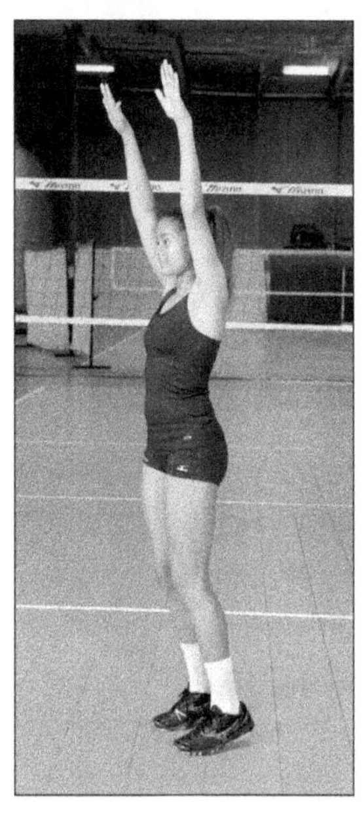

used in playing sports (think of the jump shot in basketball or spike in volleyball).

Combined with strength training, a plyometric workout is ideal for conditioning a kid for sports play and preventing injury.

Try these lower extremity and knee-protecting exercises:

Ankle bounce: Do twenty-five seconds of ankle bounce with the knees slightly bent and arms raised as you bounce up and down off the ball of the foot and toes.

Core ball hamstring curl: Assume start position as shown by lying on the floor, back of calves resting against ball (A). Lift butt off floor by lifting hips toward ceiling. Pull the ball in with your feet (B & C). Push the ball back out, return to start position and repeat. This exercise also strengths the back.

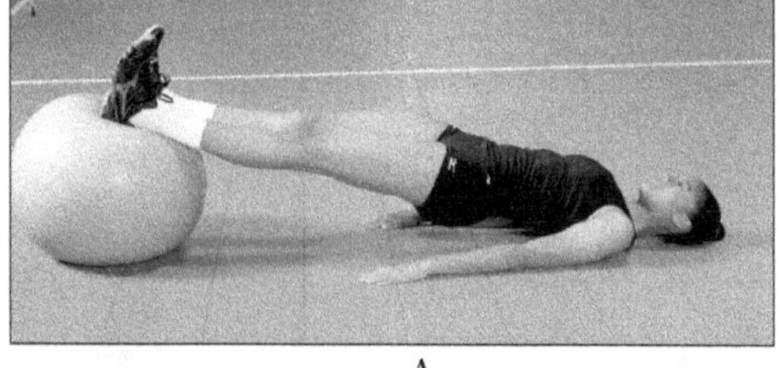

A

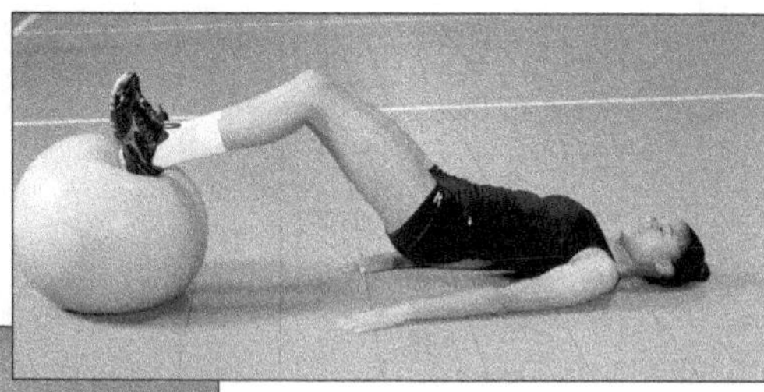

B

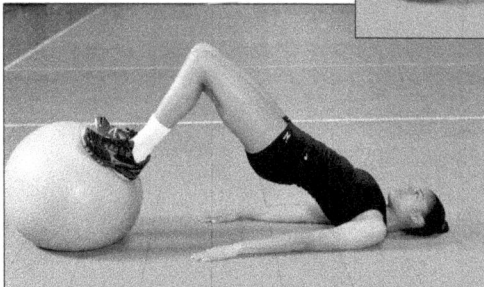

C

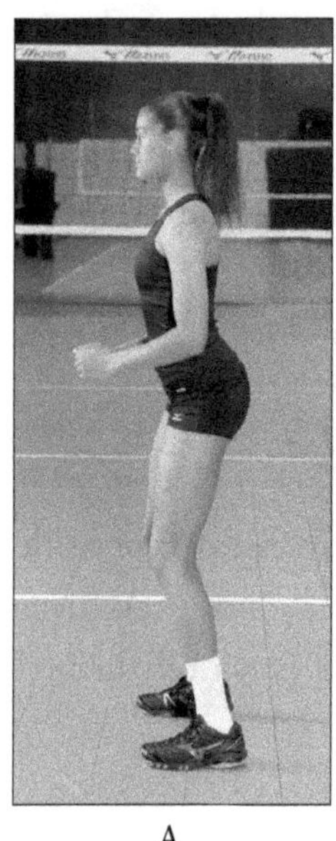

A

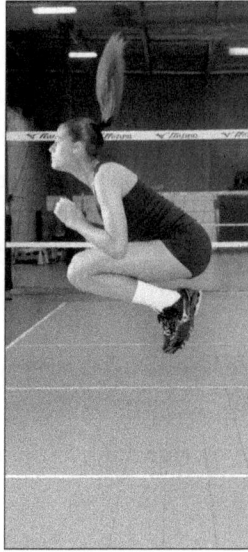

B

Tuck jump: Do twenty-five seconds of tuck jumps, jumping from the standing position (A) and bringing both knees up to the chest to the maximum height of the jump (B).

Squat jump: Do fifteen seconds of squat jumps and jump (A) with the hands in a comfortable position (B) and land in a squat position (C)A

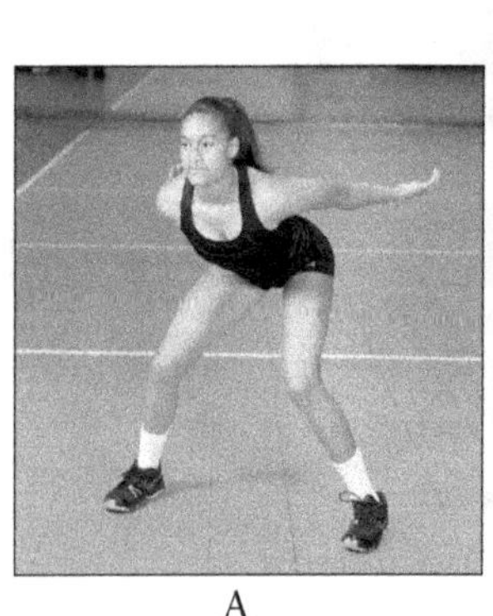

A

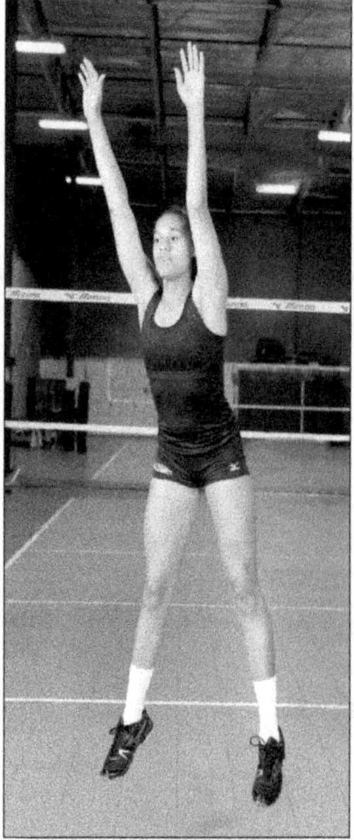

B

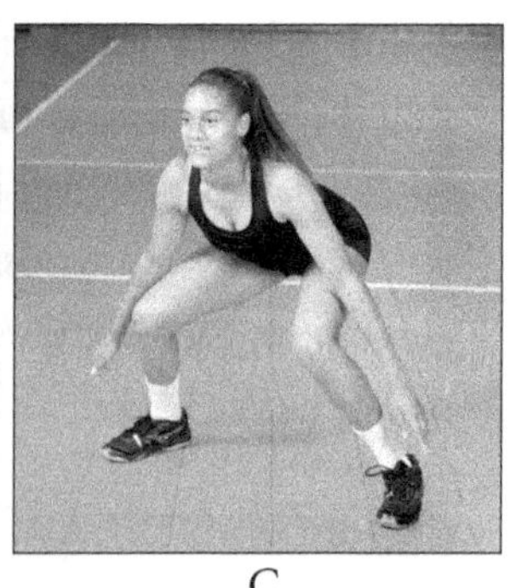

C

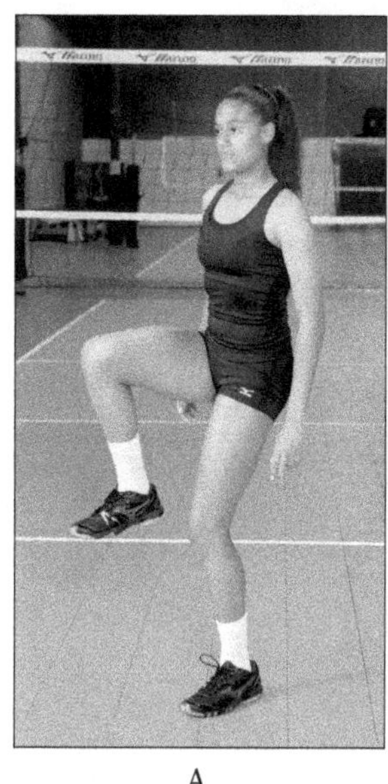

A

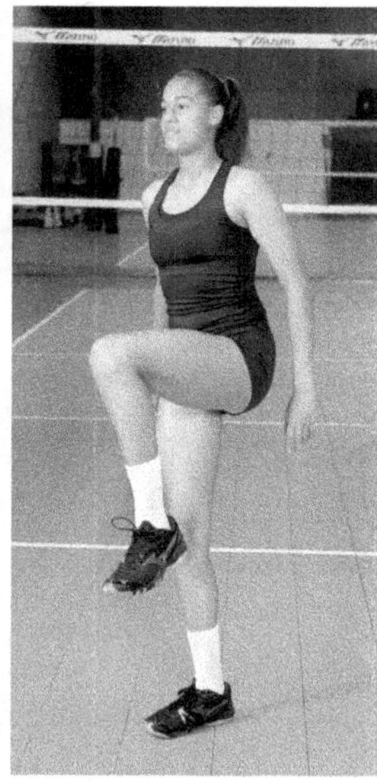

B

Bounding on the spot: For twenty-five seconds jump from one leg (A) to another (B), straight up and down, increasing the speed and the height.

180-degree squat jump: For twenty-five seconds jump off two feet (A) and turn 180 degrees in the air, (B) hold the landing for two seconds (C) and then jump again in the opposite direction.

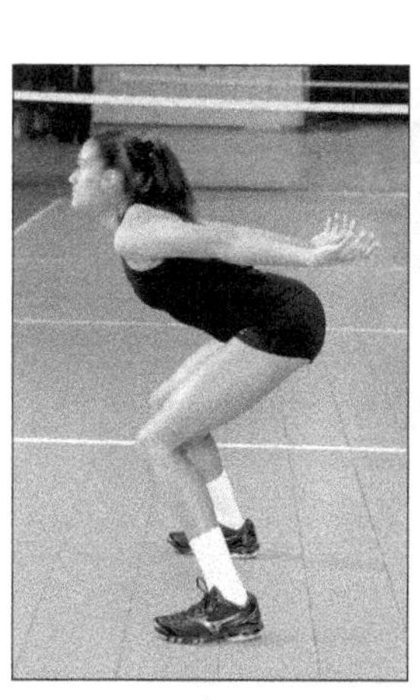

A

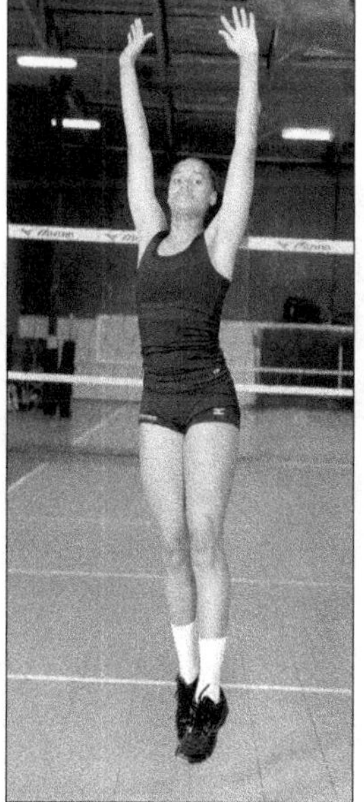

B

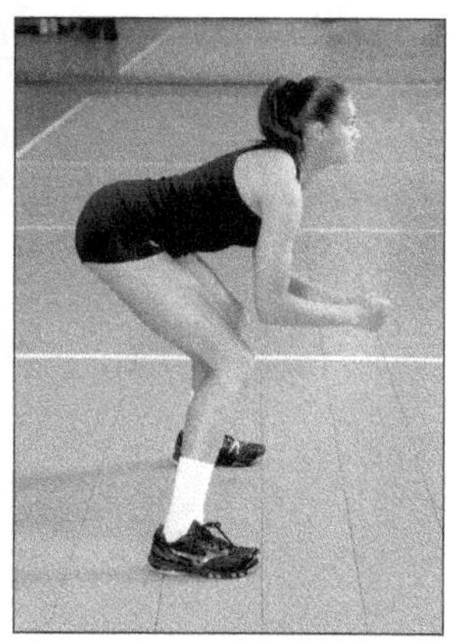

C

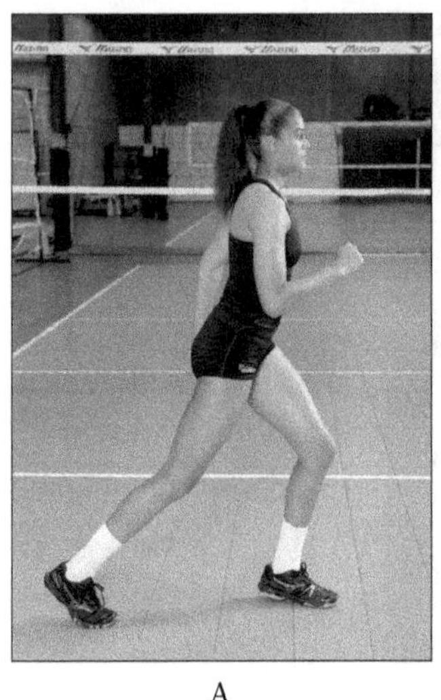

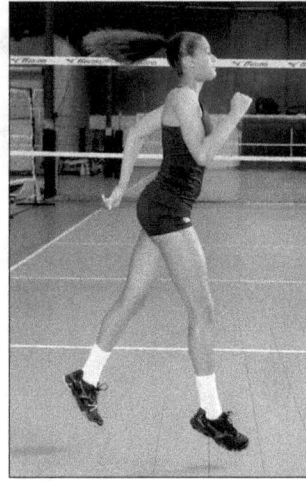

A

B

Scissor jump: Start from stride position with one foot in front of the other (A) and alternate the foot in midair (B). Do this for thirty seconds.

Bulgarian split squat: Start the exercise facing away from a bench that is about knee high and one full stride length away. Place the left foot with the laces down back on the bench (A). Bend your knee with it lined up over your right ankle until your left knee nearly touches the floor. Push back up through the heel of the right foot to straighten your right leg (B). Do eight to twelve reps (that's one set) and then switch legs. Do three sets on each side.

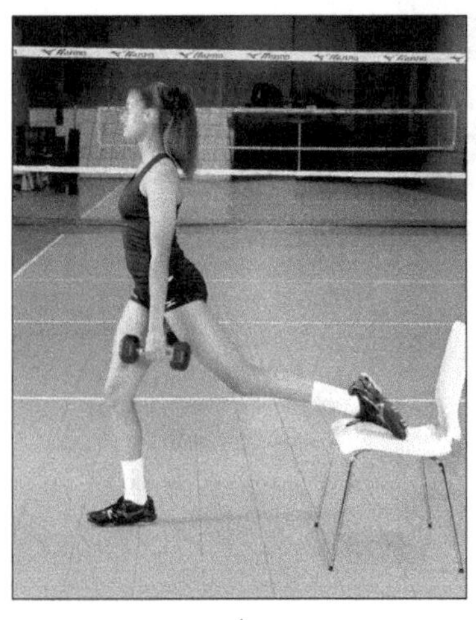

A

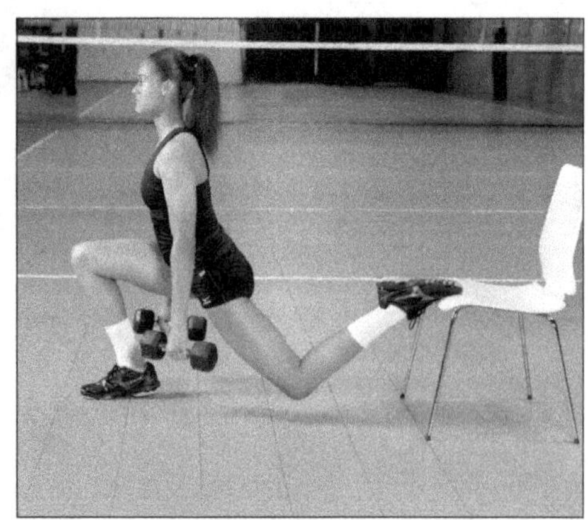

B

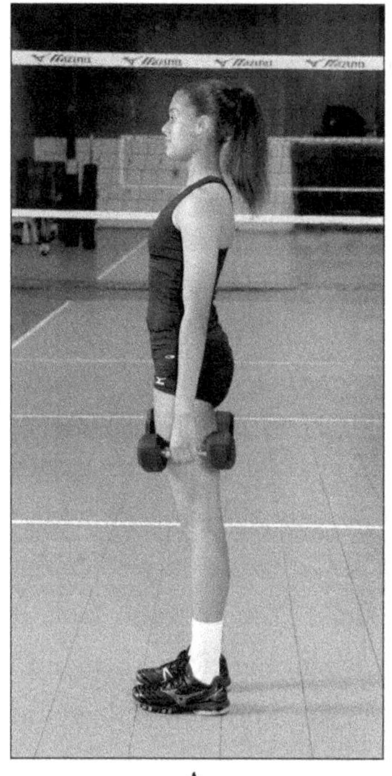

A

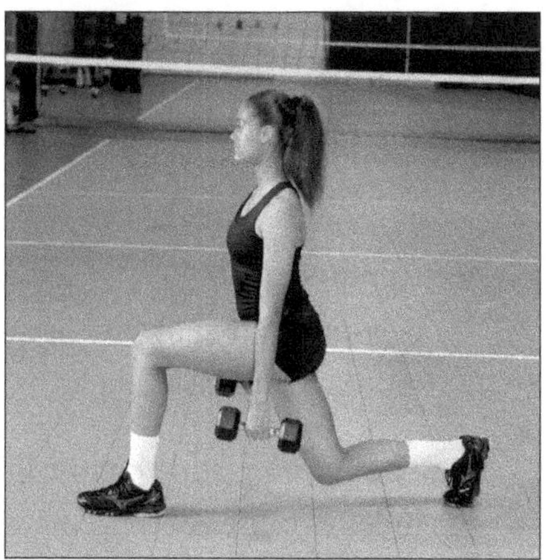

B

Reverse squat: Stand with your feet apart about as wide as your hips (A). With a five- to ten-pound dumbbell in each hand, step backward with your right foot and lower your body until the right knee is a few inches above the ground (B). Return to the start position and alternate the legs. Do three sets of eight to twelve reps.

MY MEDICAL ADVICE

- A year-round or preseason conditioning program is important.
- Weight lifting is key to prevention, and all athletes are considered beginners unless they have strength training incorporated into their program. At an early age the benefits include neuromuscular conditioning but very little addition of mass to their physique. At an older age, the mass will build, and the muscle will grow. The stronger and larger muscles can help protect the ACL of the female volleyball player, and in football players the stronger neck muscles help prevent concussion.
- If a kid is starting a new sport, the duration or distance for each sport should be advanced around 10 percent per week as tolerated.

The same with weight training. Only advance 10 percent of previously lifted weight (for example, if twenty pounds can be comfortably used on a weight machine for biceps, at fifteen reps in one set, the athlete can add two pounds the next training session).

- Appropriate protective equipment must be used. This is not negotiable. If somebody forgets his helmet, he doesn't play. No mouth guard? Go home.
- The running athlete most likely should get new shoes every 300 miles because the midsole cushioning loses its ability to absorb shock around that mileage. Mark your kids' shoes inside with a Sharpie. Note the date and then track the usage on a calendar, even with basketball and volleyball shoes. You can also look at the shoes from behind on a counter, without the kid in them, and if they lean to one side or another, they are worn out and should be replaced.
- Kids should have about one to two days off each week. Furthermore, there should be an off-season of at least four weeks that is worked into the year for each sport played. This is hard to do if your kids play club sports, which can be scheduled year-round.
- Playing another sport during the off-season is okay, especially if it uses other mechanics and muscle groups.
- Tuck your kids into bed early so they get a minimum of eight hours of sleep, especially if injured. A lot of body repair goes on at night while asleep.

INJURY REHAB: GETTING BACK IN THE GAME HEALTHY

It's all about rehab to get back into the game healthier, stronger than ever, and able to withstand regular play.

Treating the injured young athlete will require the use of a health care team. This team includes the athletic trainer, physical therapist, personal trainer, strength and conditioning coach, and doctor. And, of course, there are the parents, teammates, classmates, and family members.

Part of any return-to-play program will include a strength and conditioning program to prevent future injury. The principles of strength and conditioning explained in the previous section apply to any rehab program as well—with supervised modifications customized for the particular injury.

As part of the sports medicine team, my role as an orthopedic surgeon is often not only to treat the injury but to figure out a good program to let the young athlete continue to train without causing harm. It is important to identify the exercises that should be avoided and those that can be modified to keep the kid conditioned during the period of time he or she is out of the game and undergoing medical care.

As the treating doctor, I'll consult with physical therapists to tailor a program for each injured athlete. Expect your doctors to play a big part in designing and monitoring an effective rehab program.

I often recommend exercises such as pool running (deep water running with an aqua belt on), Pilates, riding a stationary bike, and doing core strengthening during recovery.

Every injury presents its own challenges, as does each injured kid. But here are some general observations about the various types of injuries I discussed in an earlier chapter and how to prevent them in the first place.

- Muscle strains: Compression wraps, warm-ups, and stretching after workouts and game play can help prevent muscle strains.

- Shoulder injuries: In general, instability of the shoulder can be anterior (forward) or posterior (backward). Strengthening the rotator cuff and scapular muscles may be the most important thing that the young athlete does to prevent shoulder injury (Hertling and Kessler 1996).

- Because shoulder and elbow injury are often the result of overuse and poor mechanics, care should be taken to keep an accurate pitch count and make sure a kid is not playing too long in the front row in volleyball without rotating out.

- To avoid muscle strains/sprains, warm-up is important to get the muscles warmer, more flexible, and ready for work. A jump rope or gentle jog is a good warm-up. It will help prevent injury.

- Wear proper protective gear. The biggest problem is forgetting it and not wearing it at all. The second biggest problem is wearing protective gear that does not fit or is broken. Helmets, face guards, thigh pads, ankle braces, and properly fitting shoes are important to prevent injury. The face guard will help prevent dental and eye injury in addition to facial lacerations. Well-fitted shoes will help prevent blisters, plantar fasciitis, Achilles tendinitis, and, in many cases, ankle sprains.

- Ankle sprains can be prevented in some athletes by wearing a semirigid brace. In addition, a properly fitted shoe that is not worn down on the outer sole (so it does not slide) and is not worn down on the heel (so there is still some side-to-side stability) is an asset for protecting the ankle in sports.

- Knee injuries, especially the ACL, in the female athlete may be avoided and less risky if the gluteal, core, hamstring, and quadriceps muscles are strengthened with weight training and jumping exercises such as the squat jump. Research supports doing these exercises.

- Stronger neck muscles decrease the risk for concussion. This supports the head and decreases jarring motion to some extent. Decreasing the risk for concussion has been linked to avoiding improper tackling techniques such as in the head down position. Keep your head up and be safe!

WATER, WATER, EVERYWHERE, SO DRINK IT

Kids should not wait until they are thirsty to drink. The same goes for adults. You've heard that we should all drink eight eight-ounce glasses of water every day.

Players require more (around ten glasses, unless they are very young). Most athletes do not drink enough. Dehydration is a common problem for athletes. This is made worse when a player is wearing heavy clothing and pads such as in football. The heavy clothing does not let the heat disperse and also causes increased sweating. Hard training will increase sweating, and all these factors make for fluid loss and can lead to dehydration, which means the body has lost body fluid.

Coaches must allow the athletes the opportunity to drink. The young athlete should drink before (starting about three hours before to give the water time to get into the bloodstream), during, and after practice and a game. If a practice or training session is less than one hour, water is the drink of choice. Otherwise, a sports drink can be useful, but avoid caffeine, stimulants, excess sugar, and carbonation.

As tempting as it is to grab one of those fancy "sports" drinks, your kids just need water. The athlete must drink more fluid than the average person. Water will do just as nicely as fluid replacements. The concentrations of sugar and electrolytes in sports drinks can slow down absorption in many cases. However, if the drink has a pleasant taste, the athlete will drink more fluid, and the sports drink may come in handy.

The athlete should also sip the fluid regularly during practice and on game day. Carbonated drinks will cause gas to form in the intestines, and this will slightly delay absorption. Keep in mind that the thirst mechanism is not directly proportional and timed with dehydration. If an athlete waits to drink until he or she is thirsty, then the athlete is already dehydrated. The athlete will try to play catch up with regard to fluid intake and will fail to do so.

Fluid replacement does not occur rapidly. The athlete must drink prior to the event and during the event. Drink sixteen ounces per hour for three hours prior to the game or hard practice; drink during the game and practice; drink one pint of water per pound of body weight lost, and this should occur during the six hours following the conclusion of the game or practice. Only water.

And I must caution you that those sports drinks often contain ingredients you would never want your kids drinking. They are caffeine-like substances with names such as guarana and taurine and ginseng. These stimulants can be cleverly disguised under unfamiliar names.

Why is water so important? Hard training, warm weather, and heavy clothing and pads can lead to dehydration and loss of body fluid. Dehydration can cause problems. A 3 to 4 percent body weight loss due to dehydration can result in a decrease of physical performance by 30 percent. The young athlete will lose strength, speed, stamina, and mental toughness. Over time the athlete may cramp and tire easily.

If training continues, heat-related illness may occur—starting with the least "worst," which is heat cramps, and moving quickly to life-threatening heat stroke.

Hot Weather Problems to Avoid

Athletes who start acting confused after being out in the hot sun during a game or practice may be suffering from one of these hot-weather-related problems.

Coaches and everyone else on the sidelines must be alert to the symptoms and take appropriate first aid actions:

- **Heat cramps** are painful, brief muscle cramps that occur during exercise in a hot environment. The cramps are usually felt in the calves, thighs, abdomen, or shoulders. This player should be taken into the shade or air conditioning and allowed to sip water and cool down before being sent home.
- **Heat exhaustion** occurs when the body is not able to maintain normal functions because of the excessive loss of body fluids and salts. In effect, the body is trying to protect itself from a greater rise in body temperature. The symptoms

include heavy sweating, intense thirst, dizziness, nausea, and a weak or rapid pulse. At this point, the athlete needs IV fluids (a trip to the ER). An electrolyte sports drink may help.

- **Heat stroke** is a life-threatening emergency. It is the result of the body's inability to regulate its core temperature. As the body's water and salt supplies dwindle, its temperature rises to extreme levels. The symptoms include a body temperature above 104 degrees F (although heat stroke can occur at lower body temperatures), disorientation, confusion, or coma. The skin may be hot and dry or sweaty. Time to call 911 for an ambulance.

Here's the cold, hard truth: Most athletes do not drink enough. The thirst mechanism is not directly timed with dehydration. If athletes wait to drink until they are thirsty, they are already dehydrated. Those athletes will have a hard time catching up with the thirst.

Coaches must allow athletes to drink to keep their players healthy and to maintain performance in a game. Fluid replacement does not occur rapidly. Hydration must start before a game or practice.

How Much Water Should My Child Drink?

- Before the game or practice, encourage sixteen ounces per hour for three hours prior to the activity.
- During the game or practice (small, frequent sips from a water bottle that is not shared among teammates), eight to sixteen ounces during every water break.
- After the activity, drink one pint of water per pound of body weight lost during a game or practice during the six hours following the end of the event.

If your child is dehydrated, he or she will not be able to urinate and whatever is urinated is dark. A well-hydrated child athlete should be able to urinate about every two hours, and the urine should look slightly yellow like lemonade not apple juice.

YOU REALLY ARE WHAT YOU EAT

I could write another book about what your child should be eating to fuel for sports. But that's not my area of medical specialty. I do, however, know what's best, and I'll present my checklist for healthier eating here.

- Breakfast is the most important meal. Best breakfast choices are fruit, yogurt, whole grain bread, cheese, protein shakes, eggs, meat, fish, avocado, and whole grain pancakes or waffles.
- Eat a nutritious meal two to four hours before practice or a game. Your kid needs this fuel. A sample ideal meal might be grilled chicken, grilled vegetables, whole grain bread, fruit, salad, whole grain/brown rice.
- Eat another nutritious meal one to two hours after the practice or game. This meal replenishes the lost nutrients.
- Chocolate milk has been shown to be a good fluid replacement drink after a game or practice.
- Do not skip meals.
- If you must grab and go, make sure it's a banana, apple, dried fruit, nuts, peanut butter, protein shake, or low-fat cheese. Sports bars are often no better than a Snickers.
- Avoid high fat, high sugar, and fast foods. Is it possible to make a healthy choice in the drive-through lane? Yes. Apples, single burger, milk, salad, yogurt.
- Fruits and vegetables are the best sources of carbohydrates and fiber.
- Maintain a healthy, comfortable weight. Your family doctor will have your child's health records and can track his or her weight. Be guided by the doctor's judgment based on height, weight, and growth pattern.
- Calories are necessary for top performance and mental acuity. Figure skaters, divers, gymnasts, cheerleaders, wrestlers, and runners often feel intense pressure to lose weight. If you feel your child may have an eating disorder, talk with your family doctor first for a referral to a mental health specialist/psychologist.

- Dairy products are a good source of calcium and should be included in a smart diet. Calcium is required for bone and muscle health and weight maintenance. Milk that is 2 percent is recommended for teenagers. For younger kids, whole milk is the best choice.
- Vitamin D goes hand in hand with calcium. It helps the body absorb the calcium. If your kids don't get enough vitamin D from their diet (and most don't), ask your family doctor about taking a daily vitamin that includes enough D to meet their daily requirements. Right now the recommendations from the Food and Nutrition Board are 600 IU (that's international units) daily for all of us to age seventy-one. Being in the sun helps the body make its own vitamin D (but your kids are wearing sunscreen, right? which blocks the sun's rays). Best diet sources are salmon, tuna, and fortified breakfast cereals and milk. Read labels to know.
- Supplements are not necessary, but if you want to make a protein shake, check with your doctor, trainer, or coach for a recommendation.

Sunscreen Sense

Now about that sunscreen. If your kid is playing or practicing outdoors, sunscreen is mandatory on all body parts not covered by equipment. That means face, ears, neck, hands, shins, forearms.

Here are the new rules based on updated FDA labeling for sunscreens and guidelines issued by the American Academy of Dermatology.

- You won't find *sunblock* on the labels from now on. And you won't find *waterproof* on the sunscreen labels either. Nothing blocks the sun other than clothing, and not even then.
- Look for *broad spectrum* to be protected against UVA and UVB sun rays.
- Buy *SPF 30* or higher.

- If the sunscreen is *water resistant*, you'll also see the designation 40 or 80 minutes, which is the amount of time it works before you need to reapply. No sunscreens were ever waterproof or sweat proof anyway. And not all new sunscreens are water resistant.

- Don't buy sunscreens that contain insect repellant. The AAD says you should buy two different products. Apply the insect repellant only once. The sunscreen you'll need to apply more often.

- Toss out all your outdated sunscreen lotions and tubes. The potency does expire. Start fresh every season. Read the labels. Be sun smart.

The American Academy of Dermatology recommends using an ounce (a shot glass size measures one ounce) each time you apply sunscreen to yourself (hey, you're often sitting outside too) and your team player. Apply the sunscreen before heading out to the game to allow it to sink in.

HIT THE GROUND RUNNING (IN THE RIGHT SHOES)

Does your young athlete really need a new pair of shoes for each sport? The short answer is yes. And the reason is that an appropriate shoe can prevent injuries. Plain and simple.

If your child signs up for a specific sport, he or she needs shoes designed for that sport. Sometimes the same athletic shoe can work for a couple of different sports if the function of the shoe overlaps. In other words, a Little League player can play baseball in soccer shoes at the A and AA level, but not once this kid is in the majors.

Basketball players should wear basketball shoes although any court shoe, such as tennis, would work, but those shoes break down more quickly and are not recommended. The basketball shoe provides more side-to-side stability and is built for the sudden stops and starts of basketball.

Furthermore, even basketball shoes when used for basketball will break down quickly for some kids. If they start to slide around on well-maintained courts, it is time for new shoes. If your player is not making that familiar "squeaky" sound on the court with his or her shoes, the shoes are not providing as much grip as necessary to execute the plays. Also, a slippery shoe can lead to more ankle and knee injuries.

Another exception to the sport-specific shoe rule is in football. Some football players prefer wearing a higher profile (high-top) basketball shoe—notably linemen. The higher profile shoe may provide more protection for their ankles and further stability for execution of their plays.

Some volleyball players prefer to play in basketball shoes to protect their ankles. Since the floor surface is the same—most indoor volleyball is played on basketball courts—a basketball shoe will work for volleyball. Some volleyball players feel the basketball shoe is better for side-to-side movements but cuts down on their agility in general.

Cross-training shoes can be used for tennis, but they will break down very quickly. It is recommended that there be a pivot point on the outer sole for court shoes.

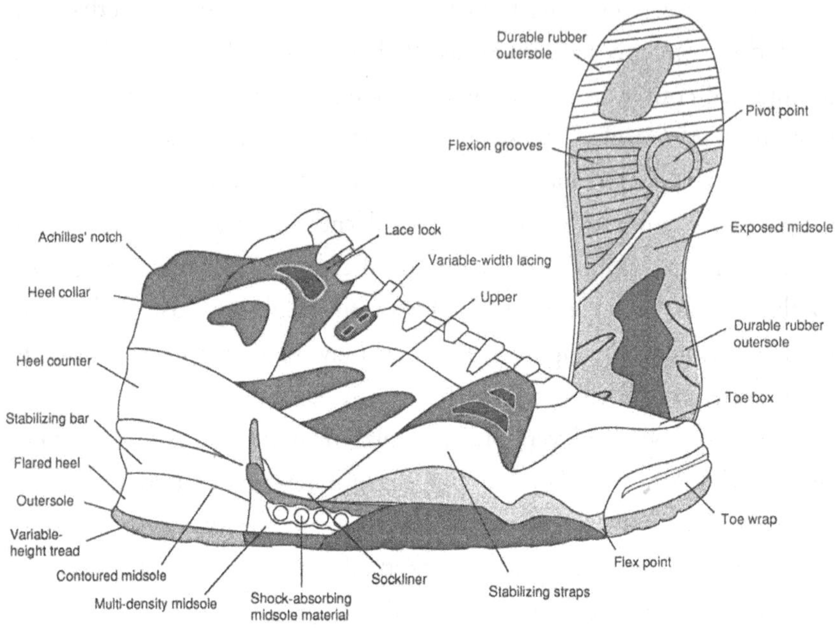

Parts of a Shoe.

Does the Shoe Fit?

In general, young children are wearing shoes that are too small. As a result of wearing too-small shoes, these kids may be at risk for developing significant foot deformities over time. A study out of Switzerland looked at 250 boys and girls from ages five to ten. The kids' indoor and outdoor shoes were measured by the researchers. They also compared the shoe measurements to the sizes given on the manufacturers' labels to see if the shoes were properly marked for size.

No surprise, most of the kids in the study were wearing the wrong size shoes: 53 percent were wearing outdoor shoes that were too small, and 13 percent were wearing outdoor shoes that were too big, and 90 percent of outdoor and indoor shoes were smaller than their marked size (American Academy of Orthopaedic Surgeons, "Don't Rely on Stated Shoe Size").

The researchers noted that the manufacturers' marked size inside the shoe almost never matched with the true size of the shoe according to industry norms as measured by the researchers.

Get the Best Fit and Other Sensible Shoe Advice

- Insist that you or the store associate measure your child's feet (both feet) every time you buy shoes for them. If one foot is larger, you'll have to buy the larger size.
- Parents need to know when the shoe fits, especially for sports shoes. Go by the fit, not by the size marked inside the shoe or on the box.
- Every parent knows kids will often outgrow their shoes before the shoes are worn out. However, once there are about three hundred miles on a shoe (or three hundred hours of practice) the cushioning properties of a shoe are usually shot anyway. (Mark the date of purchase inside the shoe with a Sharpie. It's a rough guide, but you can calculate how much practice and play time occurs using a starting date.)
- If the outer sole is worn, or the shoe tilts to one side or the other because of wear, throw the shoes away. They may cause an injury. Place the shoes on a counter top and look at them from the back and inspect the wear patterns on the outer sole.
- Kids should not wear a negative heel shoe (where the heel is lower than the toe of the shoe, like the angle on Birkenstocks or Earth shoes). This angle will put too much stress on the growth plates of the heel or the Achilles tendon. Beware that some soccer shoes are designed with a negative heel. Don't buy those brands if you have heel pain. Again, check the slope of the shoe by inspecting them on a counter top. If the heel is lower than the toe area of the shoe, then it is most likely a negative heel shoe and can cause problems in the heel.

Buying well-fitting shoes is much more than just checking the ads and comparing prices in the Sunday paper and going to your local sporting goods or athletic shoe retailer. You are making an investment in your children's feet and lowering the potential for injury.

Should you trust the advice of the shoes sales associates? Sometimes. If they work in a store that sells exclusively athletic shoes, they may have some sport-specific and shoe fitting expertise. I would be less likely to trust the advice of a shoes sales associate at one of the major discount megastores. Need I name them?

The shoe store should have appropriate devices to measure the size of the feet, and the sales associates should know how to do the measuring. Don't be swayed by a salesperson who says, "Well, he'll grow into these. Buy a half size larger." You want the shoe to fit today, not tomorrow.

You already know that both feet need to be measured. You already know that the size marked on the box may not be the size of your kid's feet. Fit is what matters. Here's a checklist to consult when you're trying on shoes for your kid's sport.

Shoe-Buying Checklist

- Shop for shoes at the end of the day, or after a practice, when the kid's feet are at the largest. Feet swell during the day and with play. Take a fresh pair of the type of socks your kid wears to play in.
- Fit to the largest foot (66% of us have feet that do not match in size).
- Try on shoes designed for the sport your child plays.
- Stand and make sure that there is one adult's thumb width from the end of the largest toe to the end of the toe box of the shoe.
- Kids should be able to freely wiggle all of their toes. There should be no slippage of the heel when walking.
- Shoes should be immediately comfortable, especially sports shoes. There is no "break-in period" for size.

- There should be no pressure points, especially where there are seams, laces, and tongues. Put your hand inside the shoe and make sure there are no prominent seams or poor construction. You'll be able to feel any rough edges.
- Fully lace the shoe for fit. Some shoes are shown with a "show lace pattern" rather than the regular crisscross pattern. Try the shoes on with the correct lacing pattern. Re-lace them yourself or ask the sales associate to do so.
- The shoe should match the shape of the foot. Have the child stand next to the shoe. The shoe should not constrict the foot.

Lacing: Do It Right the First Time

Chances are that you learned how to lace and tie your shoes in kindergarten and haven't thought about it since. Given all the differences in feet, one lacing pattern for shoes cannot fit the needs of every athlete. In fact, certain lacing patterns prevent injuries, alleviate pain, and relieve foot problems. (Adults reading this may already be wondering if their own shoes are laced properly. If your own shoes aren't feeling comfortable, you might consider changing the way they are laced.)

Follow these general lacing tips and teach your children these techniques:

- Loosen the laces as you slip into the shoes. This prevents unnecessary stress on the eyelets and the backs of the shoes. How many times do you see your kids jamming their feet into laced shoes because they're too lazy to loosen the laces? I thought so.
- Always begin at the bottom and pull the laces one set of eyelets at a time to tighten. This prevents unnecessary stress on the top eyelets and provides for a more comfortable shoe fit.
- When buying shoes, don't cringe when you see a large number of eyelets. In fact, you might want many of them because it's easier to adjust the shoe for a custom fit.

- The conventional method of lacing, crisscross to the top of the shoe, works best for the majority of athletes. Redo lacing with flat laces across the eyelets. They just do that for show in the store.
- You can adjust the lacing pattern to help the shoe fit your foot better. Following are seven lacing patterns and their uses depending on the size, shape, and anatomy of your feet.

Seven Lacing Patterns

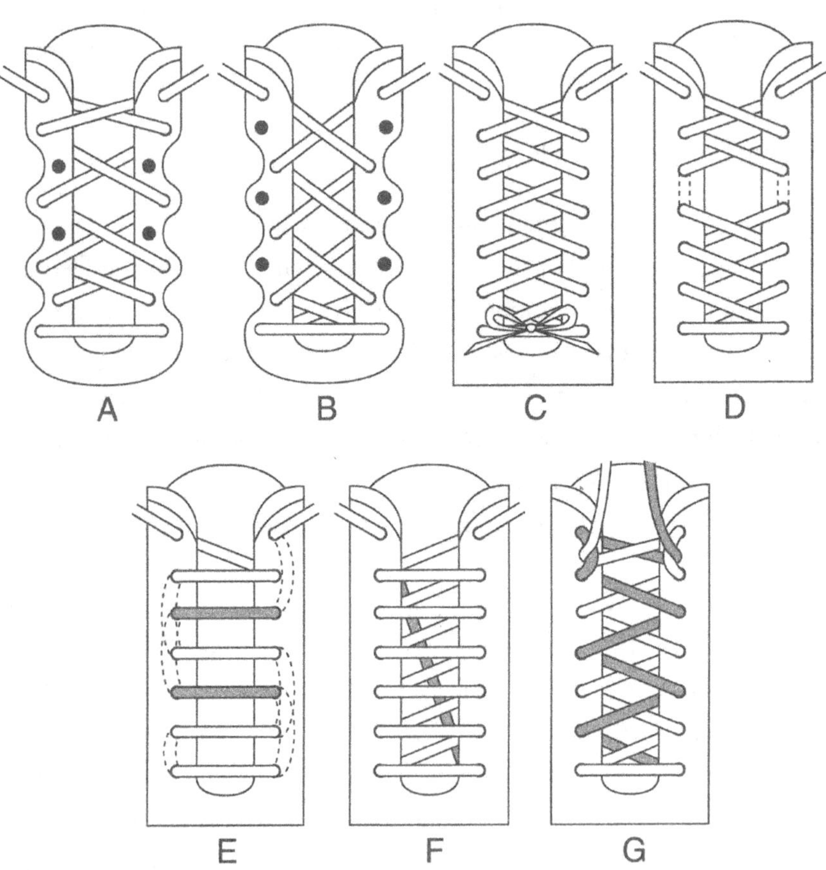

Shoe lacing patterns: The way your child laces his or her shoes will fine-tune the fit of the shoes. This may help if your child has certain problems (listed here) or if your athlete is growing or between shoe sizes.

A. For narrow feet, use the eyelets that are set wider apart on the shoe. This will bring the sides of the shoe tight together.
B. If you have wide feet, use the eyelets that are set closer to the tongue. This will have the effect of letting out the width of the shoe.
C. If you have a narrow heel and a wide foot in the front, using two sets of laces can help. Both sets of eyelets can be used, so that you can tighten the back part of the shoe and let out the front part.
D. If you have a bump on the top of your foot, or a pinched nerve or painful area, simply skip those laces that cross over this area.
E. If you have high arches, lace your shoes so that they travel in a straight line from eyelet to eyelet. If you avoid the crisscross pattern, there are no pressure points on the top of the foot.
F. If you have toe problems such as calluses, blisters, or ingrown toenails, you can lift the toe area of the shoe off this area by pulling the lace that travels directly from the toe to the top of the shoe.
G. If the shoe is slipping in the heel area or you have blisters or a bump in the heel, try this lace pattern.

A. For kids with narrow feet: If your child has a narrow foot, use the eyelets set wider apart on the shoe. This will bring up the sides of the shoe more tightly across the top of the narrow foot.

B. For kids with wide feet: If your child's feet are wide, consider using the eyelets closer to the tongue of the shoe. Use the eyelets that are closer together and this will give more width to the lacing area and have the same effect as letting out a corset.

C. For kids with a narrow heel and wide forefoot: When the ball of the foot is wide but the heel narrow, consider using two laces to get a combination fit. Use both sets of eyelets to achieve a custom fit. Use the closer set of eyelets to let out the width of the shoe at the forefoot and the wide set of eyelets to snug up the heel.

D. To address specific foot pain: If your child has a bump on the top of the foot, a high arch, a bone that sticks out, or a painful area in general, consider leaving a space in the lacing pattern to relieve pressure. Simply skip the eyelets at the point of pain. This lace pattern will increase the comfort of the shoe.

E. For the kid with high arches: Lace the shoes so that the laces travel in a straight line from eyelet to eyelet. Avoid the crisscross pattern, which can create pressure points on the top of a high arch.

F. Got toe problems? If your child has curled or bent toes, toenail problems, blisters, or calluses, you can lift the toe area off the foot by pulling on the lace that travels directly from the toe to the top of the shoe.

G. To adjust heel fit: To prevent slippage of the heel in the shoe and heel blisters, try threading the top laces through each other before tying the shoe. This will give a more snug fit to the heel.

Do Kids Need Orthotics?

Again, the simple answer is no. Most kids do not need orthotic devices.

Orthotics are inserts for the shoes that usually replace the sock liner and are designed to support the arch. These inserts are sometimes called arch supports, but they can do much more. They can be flexible, semiflexible, or rigid.

Kids who have arch strain from flat feet may need an orthotic device. If a young athlete has had stress fractures, an orthotic device may be helpful. If the player has a high arch and is getting strain or increased stress on the outside of the foot or ankle, an orthotic device may be used.

It should be noted that an orthotic device has never been shown to make any significant difference in the development of the human arch. If a young athlete has flat feet but no pain, it is of more benefit to develop the intrinsic muscles of the foot (small muscles of the foot) through a foot and toe strengthening program than to wear orthotics.

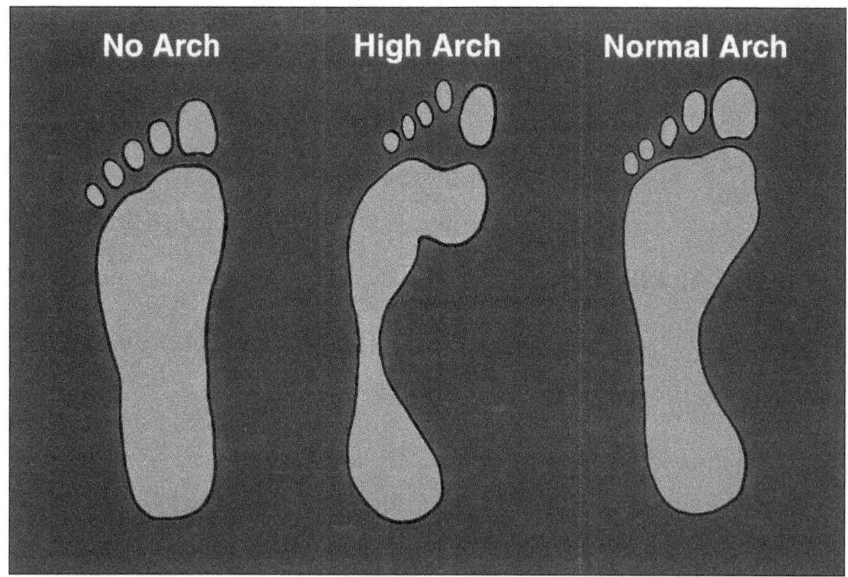

Arch type can be determined by looking at a wet footprint by the side of the pool or on a sidewalk.

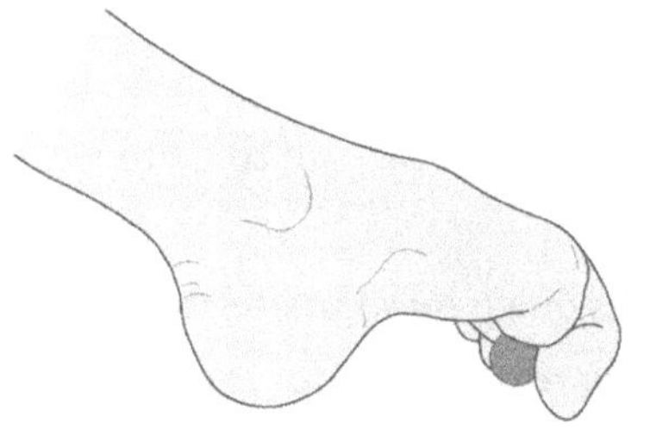

Simple exercises can be done to strengthen the toes and the arches using marbles, a towel, and a golf ball. Roll the golf ball under the arch for thirty seconds to loosen and massage the tissues. Pick up twenty marbles, one marble at a time, and transfer them from one pile to another. Do this twice. Curl a towel under your toes for two minutes.

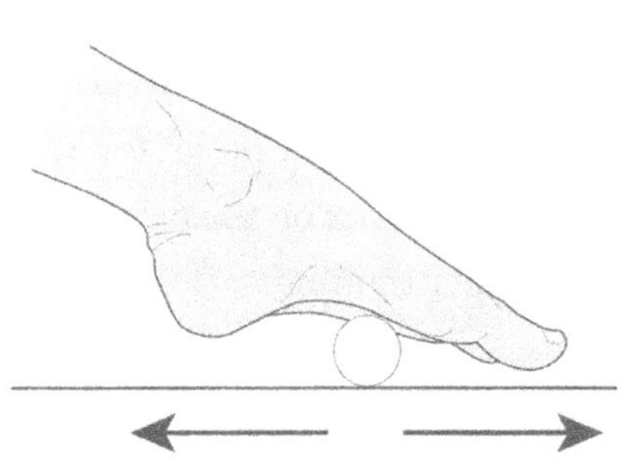

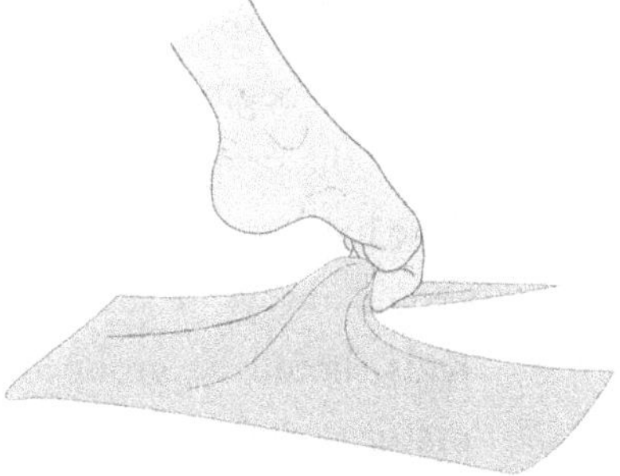

I must caution you that the long-term use of orthotic devices may even weaken the small muscles of the foot. In most cases, a young athlete does not require orthotic devices. Only a medical doctor or a doctor of podiatric medicine (DPM) should recommend orthotics (not a shoe salesperson).

MY MEDICAL ADVICE

Preventing any injury is always the priority in any sporting activity. Prevention is not difficult.

- Before starting any sport, all kids should have a physical examination by a doctor to look for any underlying medical conditions that could pose a problem on the field.
- Know the players on your kids' medical team.
- Kids should wear sport-specific, appropriate, properly fitted safety equipment when playing sports. Use the equipment for practice and games.
- Make sure appropriate first aid equipment including an AED are at the sports venue and that trained personnel are there to use it, if necessary.
- Using the right protective gear cuts down on sports-related injuries in children. However, being unaware of the risk of injury, having unavailable or inadequate equipment, and lack of funds are some of the reasons why kids do not use protective gear.
- Proper training and development of skills is the most important part of learning a sport. Proper mechanics, especially in throwing and hitting sports, should be taught at the start.
- Kids can begin strength training and conditioning. They need to know the proper technique, spotting, and weight progression. A little hard work in the gym can prevent injuries on the field. Kids should always be supervised when weight training.
- Kids should be grouped with kids who are similar in physical maturity and skill—not by age.

- Safety rules should be developed and enforced. Kids need supervision while playing sports. Kids are often unsupervised while playing sports.
- There should be no distractions on the field or bench including iPods, cell phones, food, animals, parents, friends, or other disturbances.
- Kids should drink plenty of water before, during, and after a sports event. They need to tell the coach if they are too hot. They should not play through thirst.
- Proper nutrition fuels a child's body for sports and growth. Understand the principles of healthier eating and wise food choices.
- Buy the right shoes with the right fit for the right sport. Lace them correctly.

7

Last Inning: Advice for Parents and Coaches

In the United States, around thirty million kids participate in organized sports. Some of those kids are yours. And more than 3.5 million kids will be injured playing youth sports. Chances are, those kids may be yours too. But, since so many kids do not report their injury, play through pain, or do not get treated in an ER, this number is a low estimate.

Let's hope your Little Leaguer just has a minor arm strain. Or your soccer player's ankle is merely sprained, not broken. Most injuries, fortunately, are easy-to-fix sprains and strains. Yet some sports are just more dangerous than others. And some injuries are more serious than others.

Contact sports such as football can be expected to result in a higher number of injuries than a noncontact sport such as swimming. Yet even a pickup game of basketball in the driveway has its risks. Research shows that all sports have the potential to cause injury, whether from the trauma of contact with other players or from overuse or misuse of a body part.

But let's not let the statistics discourage us from allowing our kids to play sports. On the contrary, kids who play sports are less likely to drop out of school, perhaps to get involved in gangs, and are more likely to continue on to higher education. However, it is important to prepare kids for a sport before they hit the turf, with good conditioning, drills, and skills.

Kids will have much more fun if they are playing the sport free from injury and playing with enough skill to contribute to the team. Maybe now is the time to consider the other benefits of sports such as learning teamwork, accepting defeat, building character, making friends, working hard, playing hard—and all those other life lessons that come along with playing your heart out for a team of buddies.

A continuing theme in this book is the role of supervision. Young athletes should have proper supervision, the correct equipment, and well-maintained playing surfaces. Kids also need rest and proper diet. Kids should be kids for as long as they can be and participate in many sports. Specializing too soon often leads to overuse, injury, burnout, dropout, and failure. Sports should be fun, safe, healthy, and, we all hope, enjoyed for a lifetime.

As a parent or a coach, you're in there with the team. You're on the front lines, not only signing the kids up for the sport, but also encouraging them, being a role model, attending games, driving to tournaments, and providing a positive experience. Kids benefit from their parents, and coaches, setting good examples, teaching skills, enjoying the sport, and providing support (without coddling or getting overinvolved in winning). Kids who are enjoying their sport, and not made miserable by poor behavior on the part of the adults, are much more likely to stay in the game and even go on to professional careers in sports.

SHOULD KIDS SPECIALIZE?

Parents seem more eager than ever to fast-track their kids into one sport. They may be doing more harm than good, as overuse injuries can be a direct result of specialization, especially too soon during a child's mental and physical development.

If a kid suffers an overuse injury at an early age, especially in throwing and hitting sports, that kid usually does not make it to the higher levels of play.

According to Jim Andrews, young pitchers who throw eighty or more pitches a game increase their risk of injury by 360 percent. Those who pitch more than eight months in a year increase their injury risk by 500 percent.

Those who pitch, ignoring fatigue and overuse, increase their risk of injury by 3,600 percent (Weisenberger 2011; Flesig et al. 2009).

Keep in mind that, despite a pitch count, practice throws are not counted. Therefore, the pitch count only reflects the game pitches and does not reflect practice or the "speed revolution."

There are some major shifts in the way kids (and adults) approach the game at every level. Part of the revolution is that kids are bigger and stronger than ever before. They can hit and throw harder and faster than ever before. The stress that goes through the shoulder joint with pitching reaches an all-time high when the pitcher is throwing a fastball. The shoulder goes about as fast as any human joint can go when a kid is firing off a fastball.

I've seen iPhone apps on which Little League parents can track how fast their ten-year-old is throwing. Today's young pitchers are being raised in a culture of the fastball. The coaches and pitchers are obsessed with velocity. Kids and their coaches want to work on throwing the ball as hard as they can. This results in tremendous stress on the shoulder joint. Of course, intensity is not reflected in the pitch count, but it does increase the risk for an overuse injury.

The majority of players in the NBA, according to a 2011 ESPN broadcast, played two sports in high school. Many played three. Of course, the majority of these players were behemoths who could literally jump out of the gym. They have something you cannot teach or coach: they have size.

Still, kids are getting bigger, compared to several decades ago. According to the CDC, the American adult is more than one inch taller and about twenty-five pounds heavier than the average adult in 1960 (CDC, National Health Examination and the National Health and Nutrition Examinations Surveys between 1960 and 2002). What does this mean for our purposes here?

- A fifteen-year-old boy in 1966 weighed 135.5 pounds, and by 2002, the average weight increased to 150.3 pounds.

- A fifteen-year-old girl weighed 124.2 pounds on average in 1966, and by 2002 the average girl weighed 134.4 pounds.
- The average weight for a ten-year-old boy in 1963 was 74.2 pounds, and by 2002 the average weight was 85 pounds.
- The average weight for a ten-year-old girl in 1963 was 77.4 pounds, and by 2002 it was 88 pounds.
- The average height of a fifteen-year-old boy in 1966 was 67.5 inches and by 2002 it was 68.4 inches.
- The average height of a fifteen-year-old girl in 1966 was 63.9 inches, and by 2002 it was about the same.
- The average height of a ten-year-old boy in 1963 was 55.2 inches, and by 2002 it was 55.7 inches.
- The average height of a ten-year-old girl in 1963 was 55.5 inches, and by 2002 was 56.4 inches.

Yes, there is an obesity problem among kids and adults in our country, but that doesn't account for the gains in height over the same period of time.

When it comes to preventing injury, I recommend your child participate in a variety of athletic activities. More than one sports activity allows for more balanced muscle development, more fun, and less burnout, and decreases the risk of overuse injury because each sport uses highly specific muscles and nerves.

On a practical level, some sports just seem to go together such as basketball and volleyball, basketball and track/field, basketball and football, and, in the case of Michael Jordan, basketball and baseball. You rarely see basketball and golf, or football and swimming, yet these probably would be good combinations because they stress completely different muscles groups.

I have overheard more than one parent say to a kid, "You need to pick a sport. If you try to be good at more than one sport, you will end up not being very good at either."

Nothing could be further from the truth. Especially when the kid is ten years old!

If I had my way, kids would not specialize until their senior year in high school. Since that will never happen in today's intense world of competition to get a spot on a college-level team, we need to take a more practical approach. If a child specializes at an early age, it is imperative that he or she also receives a good overall strength and conditioning program. That program should include cardio, flexibility, core strengthening (especially the pelvis), balance work, quick footwork, and age-appropriate strength training.

THE MENTAL GAME

Since there are only a handful of middle schools with well-organized team sports, most of the pre–high-school training and sports participation takes place in club sports or youth leagues.

A sound sports program, like many of these, will provide an environment where kids can develop physically and emotionally. And by emotionally, I mean the mental aspect of sports. It's tricky.

After passion, the mental "game" is probably the most important X factor. The young athlete needs to not only develop self-confidence but also focus on mental toughness. This is hard to accomplish with an immature athlete. Especially after an injury, kids question their confidence in their athletic ability. If there has been a reinjury or multiple injuries, the player begins to think he or she is fragile.

I have had more than one player tell me that he or she can see the coaches and teachers roll their eyes when the student appears in yet another cast. One very athletic basketball player, at the high school level, told me he thought the coach hated him because he was injured so often (two ankle injuries, two jumper's knees, and one concussion).

But it was apparent that the coach was just as frustrated as the injured player. Even when the ankle was fully healed, from the point of view of the team doctor, the player did not trust his ankle. From the point of view of the coach, he saw a great player with no confidence. It was time for a sports psychologist to step in.

Some kids have negative experiences and sustain real emotional injury. Some physical injuries are caused by emotional responses from the players themselves. One very talented freshman basketball player who could dunk in the eighth grade was upset from missing an easy shot during a practice and punched the gym wall as hard as he could with his fist.

The school had been built in 1950. The solid building and gym wall were made of exposed brick. Guess what? He not only fractured three metacarpal bones but dislocated them as well. He required surgery and was out for the majority of the season.

He was a freshman playing on the varsity team and felt that he had to be perfect to gain respect from the bench—and took himself out with a stupid act. This very talented player (possible D-1 level) has subsequently had recurrent jumper's knee and chronic tendinitis in the ankle. He is counting on the club season to get his recognition.

LET'S GET MOTIVATED

Motivation is a key factor in a kid staying with a sport and athletics, especially after an injury. Some coaches feel that each practice is a survival test. There are coaches who speak to their players in a way that would get them fired in any other job. Coaches have been caught on iPhone cameras insulting players, throwing balls at them, pushing them, punching them, cursing at them, and in general "going off" on the players. These videos look like the "before" videos for the movie *Anger Management.*

There are extreme examples where the coaches end up getting fired. But more commonly an overly critical coach leaves the players with the feeling that they are getting criticized more than coached. An injury may then shake the confidence of a young player.

Some kids may be really sensitive to criticism and comments after an injury. There are plenty of stories about coaches who tell players that they had better be in the hospital or dead to miss a practice.

It has been noted that playing sports is like war. The athlete is sent out to "subdue one's opponent through physical and mental force—without killing them. War is, of course, body bags" (Farrey 2003). A sport is, obviously, not war. A sport is supposed to be fun (at least most of the time). And if your kid is not having fun, perhaps he or she needs to move on to another sport, team, coach, or pursuit.

A group based at Stanford University called the PCA (Positive Coaching Alliance) promotes the "Magic Ratio" for coaching. The Magic Ratio recommends that there be five times more positive comments than negative in coaching (gestures included) such as "good job," "great pass," "nice block," a nod of the head, or a single positive word (Positive Coaching Alliance).

Athletes have, according to the Stanford group, an emotional tank that needs to be filled. I think that there is no firm ratio, but rather, the need for positive feedback on an intermittent basis, just so the kid doesn't think every word out of the coach's mouth is negative.

But criticism is the job of the coach. He or she only has one minute (or less) during a timeout to tell you what to do and how to improve. The coach does not have time to make players feel good about themselves. Players need to develop the skills and mental toughness to motivate themselves, remain confident, maintain self-esteem, and feel ready.

Behavioral science supports the thinking that positive intermittent reinforcement is a stronger behavioral tool than criticism (Skinner 1956). Good coaching offers criticism and tells a player what he or she is doing wrong, if it is honest. But it is just as important to develop confidence in a player with positive praise as well as promoting athletic talent.

Kobe Bryant noted that positive coaching is like "the force … like a Jedi, and he can sense his way through things."

The PCA notes that there are over four million coaches in the United States for youth sports. Few of those coaches have had any formal training. The majority are volunteers. Many of these coaches get their "training" from observing other coaches and coaches on TV. Sad to say, some of the coaching on TV has been downright horrible; coaches and athletic directors are getting fired and rightly so.

John Wooden taught that success was in the little things and would spend his first day teaching his players how to put on their shoes and socks so they would not get blisters. He had them work on the fundamentals, teamwork, effort, and character. A kid who plays for the team is better than a "great player."

Parents can monitor the coaching by going to practice and games. There is a fine (maybe not that fine) line, however, between interfering with the coaching versus exhibiting good parenting skills—being a helicopter parent versus being an objective observer, allowing the coach to control practice versus being an advocate (zealot) for your kid, and judging perceived "unfairness" versus praising a good coaching decision.

An element of trust needs to be observed among the kid, coach, and the parents. Just because a coach is not nice does not mean he or she is a bad coach. The last thing a young athlete needs, especially after a loss, is for the parent to lecture him or her on game strategy and technique. Please leave that to the coach. As a parent you need to encourage your athlete and show empathy and understanding.

Our kids are athletes. Athletes are under stress. Athletes can have periods of doubt. Kids, especially growing children, are also under stress. It would be ideal to have a relationship between the parents and the child that allows for open discussions about the stress of competition, school, relationships, growth, and self-worth. If you do have that kind of relationship with your children, you're lucky.

Sometimes it is just easier for a child to open up to a professional who has the experience to advise him or her. A sports psychologist is a type of trainer. He or she is expensive but is a tool that is often ignored in kids' sports. Not every kid needs a sports psychologist to learn how to be mentally tough. Some kids just start out that way, but some young athletes need a guide.

The coach can teach your kid how to play the game—kick, throw, jump, swing, shoot— and can advise on technical skills and conditioning routines. They do not, as a general rule, teach mental toughness. Mental toughness may just be the X factor in getting to the next level of play and having a winning season.

Have you ever seen a player freeze and not be able to do a routine or shoot a basket that they have done over a hundred times in practice? This is a mental block, most of the time. The young athlete who wants success in sports needs to face the fears, maintain a positive attitude in the face of obstacles, deal with the adversities, and not get "freaked out" by the game (performance anxiety). And perhaps most important, the kid cannot fear failing.

Some young athletes get obsessed with failing or messing up. Perfection is not the goal in sports. The goal in sports is to be the best you can be. All successful athletes have some failures (more than you think) under their belt. There are techniques that will help the young athlete through sports and all aspects of life, such as visualization, positive self-talk, breathing techniques, relaxation, meditation, and learning how to keep the mind calm and focused.

Kids should be taught how to overcome mental blocks by first recognizing that there is the conscious (cognitive) mind and the unconscious (automatic) mind. The unconscious mind is a hard one to manipulate. The conscious mind can be helped by a sports psychologist, parent, teacher, or coach who can help the student athlete learn how to give directions to the unconscious mind. The goal is to be focused, calm, determined, and confident under pressure.

I do believe that mental toughness can be taught. Keep in mind that most kids start out loving their sport. When it becomes a source of anxiety and stress, it is time to teach (or get help with) mental toughness or perhaps look for another sport or join the band. If the game gets too serious at too young an age, there is a huge risk for burnout and leaving the sport for good.

Sports devotees have become obsessed with velocity, speed, size, strength, and performance—in all sports. Part of this culture of sports intensity and "enhanced" performance comes from television and video games where children are watching their sports heroes perform amazing, superhuman in some cases, feats. They also see spectacular wipeouts, but the hero is the super fit athlete.

Don't get me wrong, I think athletes make great role models for kids because they make a living being fit, healthy, strong, and disciplined. A great role model should be great on and off the playing field. As a general rule, athletes and the athletic lifestyle are admirable examples of how your kids can love to play, love life, and avoid injury.

Acknowledgments

To Keith S. Feder, MD, orthopedic surgeon; West Coast Sports Medicine Foundation Sports Medicine Fellowship director; assistant clinical professor orthopedic surgery, UCLA; founder/board member, West Coast Sports Medicine Foundation; and consultant to the Long Beach Ice Dogs, Dew Tour, USTA, AVP, USA Weight Lifting, and USA Volleyball. He contributed high-level expertise about sports injuries as a physician and as an elite-level athlete himself. He is also my husband, who supported me and our son Jacob through the long and countless hours of research, revisions, fact-checking, and interviews. Thank you!

Richard "Ricky" Feder—my ten-year-old son, who is also a blue belt in karate, Little League power hitter, and all-around powerful positive and wonderful kid—was an inspiration on the field and allowed me to sit in my big club-size lawn chair on those sunny Little League fields for many hours. I gathered as much information on the sidelines as in any textbook or journal article.

Elisabeth "Betty" Frey, my ninety-year-old mother, who is also a former honors English teacher at Carson High School. She has a master's degree in English from USC and is a wonderful writer who taught me to "talk to the page." I love you.

Scott and James Perkins, my nephews, who provided us access to many friends with soccer injuries.

Mathew Culp, my nephew, who had a contact page full of injured fellow football players.

And to all the injured "warriors" who allowed us to interview them for these pages.

May they play again!

Glossary

abduction: Refers to the mechanical movement of the arm or leg (limbs) laterally and moving away from the midline of the body. **Adduction** is the mechanical movement of the limbs medially and toward the midline of the body.

Achilles tendon: A tendon anatomically located in the posterior, or back part, of the lower leg made of white fibrous cords, which serves to connect the calf muscles and the heel bone.

ACL (anterior cruciate ligament): A major ligament located in the front and interior of the knee made of connective tissue that acts to provide stability to the surrounding knee joint. Sports injuries to this ligament are usually a direct result of the foot planting and then the knee twists.

anterior: An anatomy term referring to the structural position of the body understood to mean directed forward or in front. The opposite is posterior or back.

apophysis: A normal type of protuberance (a bulge or lump) involving bone tissue formation originating from a growth center, which can later fuse to neighboring bone.

articular cartilage: Made of collagen and water, which surrounds the bones at the joints and found between the bones of any joint in the body. The articular cartilage reduces friction and distributes load-bearing pressure. It provides a smooth gliding surface to joints.

bone scan: An imaging procedure that requires the patient to be injected with radioactive tracer that will visually highlight abnormalities and aid in the diagnosis of fractures not seen under regular x-rays. In areas of fractures, the injured area will absorb the tracer and will appear bright.

cartilage: This material consists of flexible connective tissue more rigid in structure than muscles and made of collagen fibers, ground substance, and water. Cartilage serves to provide structure for surrounding tissues and organs, and cushions joints. The three types of cartilage are hyaline, elastic, and fibrocartilage. Hyaline cartilage can be found lining the bones where joints are located and is also called articular cartilage. Fibrocartilage connects bones to neighboring tendons and ligaments.

concussion: A temporary loss of function of the brain due to the head receiving impact from an object or the ground with violent movement. The consequence of brain injury can lead to short-term behavioral changes, cognitive loss, emotional unstableness, and sensory impairments. Concussions can lead to long-term problems in some cases.

core muscles: A network of muscles that incorporate all the physical functions of the abdomen (belly), midback, and lower back and secondarily involve the use of the neck, shoulders, and hips.

core strength: Quantitatively measures a person's physical ability to perform exercises adequately that target the core muscles of the body.

core strengthening: Activity that promotes the core muscles working together to stabilize, promote balance, increase endurance, and keep the pelvis and the spine flexible and strong.

cruciate ligament: Mainly in areas of the body where joints can be found that structurally forms the letter X. The cruciate ligaments in the knee are the anterior and posterior cruciate ligaments. The cruciate ligaments act to physically hinder any rotational movement of the knee and prevent forward movement of the lower leg connected to the femur (thighbone).

CT (computed tomography): An x-ray procedure that uses cross-sectional imaging of isolated areas of the body. Patients lie down while a rotating machine captures a segment of the body in two-dimensional or three-dimensional images utilizing a combination of different cross-sectional angles. This technique provides images that help with diagnosis of disease, fractures, and abnormalities.

epicondyle: An epicondyle is a small and round prominence located on or above the condyle of a bone. It functions as an area of attachment for ligaments, tendons, and muscles. The epicondyle in the elbow is commonly injured in sports.

epiphysis: An epiphysis is part of the round end of the long bone filled with red bone marrow and erythrocytes (red blood cells). This region of the bone is covered with articular cartilage. This is a part of a bone.

external rotation: Rotational movement away from the midline or center of the body.

femur: A bone commonly identified as the thighbone. The head of the femur is attached to the pelvic bone, and the lower part makes up part of the knee joint.

fibula: This bone is located next to the tibia of the lower leg and the smaller bone on the outside of the ankle. The fibula is the narrow bone in the lower leg.

fracture: An injury that involves the breaking of a bone. This can be a result of disease, violence, or repetitive stress on a bone.

glenohumeral joint: A joint identified as the shoulder joint. The glenohumeral joint works with the rotator cuff muscles and consists of the humeral head of the upper arm joining to the socket in the scapula, known as the glenoid. This joint is an example of a ball and socket joint, which allows various movements such as rotation, flexion, extension, abduction, and adduction of the arms.

glenoid fossa: Glenoid fossa is part of the scapula forming the hollow part of the socket for the head of a humerus to fit into.

glenoid labrum: This material is a fibrocartilage that surrounds the glenoid fossa located in the shoulder. It works to deepen the "socket" of the shoulder joint.

growth plate: Also known as epiphyseal plate, is the area where growth in the length of the bones occurs through the multiplication of specialized cartilage cells.

humeral head: A large, rounded end of the humerus that makes up the upper arm and makes up the ball part of the ball and socket shoulder joint.

humerus: A long bone in the upper arm anatomically positioned between the shoulder and elbow.

juvenile kyphosis (Scheuermann's disease): A physical deformity seen in prepubescent children who experience abnormal curvature of the thoracic spine. This condition may require medical intervention through bracing, surgery, or chiropractic treatments. The spine appears to be bent forward.

lateral: An anatomical term referring to the position of the body farthest from the midline of the body or toward the outside.

LCL (lateral collateral ligament): A ligament farthest from the middle of the knee made up of thin connective tissue. This ligament is on the lateral aspect, or outside, of the knee. This ligament functions to stabilize the knee through a full range of motion, and the ligament is located where the femur and fibula meet.

ligament: Fibrous tissue responsible for linking bones to adjacent bones.

lumbar spine: The lower part of the spine labeled L1 through L5, which functions to protect the spinal cord. The lumbar vertebrae lie below the rib cage and above the pelvis.

MCL (medial collateral ligament): One of four major ligaments in the knee and found on the inner side of the knee joint. The MCL plays a key role in the stability of the knee, which keeps the knee from moving medially, or collapsing inward.

medial: An anatomical term used to refer to the center of the body or toward the middle.

meniscus: A cartilage component of the knee joint that acts to alleviate stress from the femur (thighbone) acting on the tibia of the lower leg. The meniscus is shaped like a washer.

MRI (magnetic resonance imaging): This procedure utilizes magnetic fields to create two-dimensional or three-dimensional depictions of the body. MRI can provide visuals of the brain, heart, muscles, and soft tissues such as ligaments better than CT scans or x-rays. MRI uses high-powered magnets to produce an image. No radiation is used.

Osgood-Schlatter disease: A condition that produces an inflamed bump on the patellar ligament located at the upper shinbone (tibia). This syndrome occurs during the time of puberty of both boys and girls but is more prevalent in male adolescents. The disease is brought on by repeated injury and overuse of the injured area. Small bumps located below the knee are characteristic features of the disease. It is sometimes referred to as "jumper's knee."

osteochondritis dissecans (OCD): A joint condition involving the death of tissues of cartilage and underlying bone due to decreased blood flow. A section of the bone separates from the rest of the bone. Young males and females who are physically active can experience this medical condition, but OCD is more common in males than females. The disease is common in the knees, hips, and ankles, and recovery without intervention is commonly seen in teens.

patella: The patella, or kneecap, is located in the front of the knee and is considered part of the knee joint together with the thighbone and shinbone, where they meet.

patella tendon: A tendon that attaches the front of the kneecap to the front of the shinbone, or tibia, of the lower leg. A breakage, or rupture, of the patella tendon causes the patella to move up the thighbone.

posterior: Refers to the anatomical position of the body located behind or toward the rear.

PRICE MM: Acronym for Protect, Rest, Ice, Compression, Elevation, Modalities, and Medication as immediate and home treatment for some sports injuries.

radius: A major bone located in the forearm made up of a small proximal end, part of the elbow, a body and a distal end, which is large in diameter and is part of the wrist. The radius is positioned lateral to the ulna, and located between the elbow and thumb side of the wrist. The radius can rotate around the ulna.

rotator cuff: A group of muscles that stabilizes and allows the shoulder joint to rotate. The muscles involved are the Teres minor, Infraspinatus, Supraspinatus, and Subscapularis.

Salter-Harris Classification: An injury to the growth plate of the bone seen in growing children. This classification can grade severity of the injury.

Sports Concussion Assessment Tool 2 and 3 (SCAT 2 and 3): A standardized test used to evaluate the severity of a concussion for athletes. This allows physicians and health professionals to provide appropriate treatments based on a quantitative analysis of a concussion.

spondylolysis: This condition, which occurs almost exclusively in adolescents, is a special type of stress fracture in the vertebrae and produces lower back pain. The injury is commonly seen in athletes who bend backward at the spine such as in gymnastics, volleyball, and basketball.

sprain: An injury to a ligament, in various degrees.

Tanner Stages (Scale): A scale that quantifies the development of children's growth based on gender-specific primary and secondary physical characteristics.

tendon: A type of connective tissue responsible for attaching muscles to bones.

tibia (shinbone): The second largest bone in the human body, located medially in the lower leg. The tibia's upper portion is found below the knee, and the lower portion is above the ankle.

ulna: A long bone found in the medial side of the forearm in humans that supports the elbow structure. The ulna extends from the elbow joint, where it articulates with the humerus, all the way to the little finger side of the wrist joint.

valgus: An orthopedic term that described the outward angle of the distal end of bones or joints. This is prevalent in areas of the hip, knee, and foot of the human body. An example is valgus of the knees, or knocked knees. The joint will appear to collapse inward when in valgus.

varus: An orthopedic term that refers to distal segments of bones or joints being inwardly angled. An example is varus of the knees, or bowed legs. The joint will appear to collapse outward when in varus.

Works Cited

American Academy of Orthopaedic Surgeons. "Don't Rely on Stated Shoe Size." Accessed June 1, 2013. http://www.aaos.org/news/aaosnow/mar09/clinical5.asp.

American Academy of Orthopedic Surgeons. "Preserving the Future of Sport: From Prevention to Treatment of Youth Overuse Sports Injuries." Presented at the AOSSM Annual Meeting Pre-Conference Program, Keystone, Colorado, 2009.

American Academy of Pediatrics. Accessed June 1, 2013. http://www.aap.org.

American Association of Cheerleading Coaches and Administrators. Accessed June 1, 2013. http://www.aacca.org.

Aury, M. et al. "Summary and Agreement Statement of the First International Conference on Concussion in Sport, Vienna 2001." *Clinical Journal of Sports Medicine* 12 (January 2002): 6–11.

Bachner-Melman, R., A. Zohar, R. Ebstein et al. "How Anorexic-like Are the Symptom and Personality Profiles of Aesthetic Athletes?" *Medicine & Science in Sports & Exercise* 38 (2006): 628–36.

Belson, Ken. "A 5-Concussion Pee Wee Game Leads to Penalties for the Adults." *The New York Times,* Oct. 23, 2012.

Beighton, P.H., L. Solomon, and C.L. Soskolne. "Atricular Mobility in an African Population." *Annals of the Rheumatic Diseases* 32 (1973): 413–27.

Buddle, Renee Blisard. "Former NFL Players with More Concussions Have Greater Risk of Developing Depression." *Orthopedics Today*, December 2012.

Carry, P.M. et al. "Adolescent Patellofemoral Pain: A Review of Evidence for the Role of Lower Extremity Biomechanics and Core Instability." *Orthopedics* 33 (July 2010): 498–507.

Centers for Disease Control and Prevention (CDC). "Heads Up: Concussion in Youth Sports." Accessed June 1, 2013. http://www.cdc.gov/ConcussionInYouthSports.

Centers for Disease Control and Prevention. "Mean Body Weight, Height and Body Mass Index, United States, 1960–2002." October 27, 2004. Accessed June 1, 2013. http://www.cdc.gov/nchs/data/ad/ad347.pdf.

Centers for Disease Control and Prevention. Morbidity and Mortality Weekly Report. "Mental Health Surveillance Among Children–United States, 2005–2011." Accessed June 1, 2013. http://www.cdc.gov/mmwr/preview/mmwrhtml/su6202a1.htm.

Centers for Disease Control and Prevention. "NIOSH FACTS, NFL Mortality Study." January 1994. Accessed June 1, 2013. http://www.cdc.gov/niosh/pdfs/nflfactsheet.pdf.

Chhabra, A., "Challenges in the Sideline Management of Concussion." Presented at the American Orthopaedic Society for Sports Medicine (AOSSM), 2011 Annual Meeting, San Diego, CA, July 7–10, 2011.

Committee on Sports Medicine and Fitness, 2000–2001. Reginald L. Washington, MD, Chairperson.

Consumer Product Safety Commission. "National Electronic Injury Surveillance System." Accessed June 1, 2013. http://www.cpsc.gov.

Corbett, Jim. "NFL Passes New Helmet Rule, Eliminates 'Tuck Rule.'" *USA Today Sports,* March 20, 2013.

Daneshvar, D.H., C.U. Nowinski, A.C. McKee, and R.C. Cantu. "The Epidemiology of Sports-Related Concussion." *Clinics in Sports Medicine* 30 (January 2011): 1–17.

Durant, S. "Raising Successful and Emotionally Healthy Children in a Competitive World." *Independent School* 66 (2007): 116.

Ewing, M.E. and V. Sefeldt. "Participation and Attrition Patterns in American Agency-Sponsored Youth Sports." In *Children and Youth in Sports,* edited by F.C. Small and R.E. Smith. Madison, WI: Brown & Benchmark, 1996.

Faigenbaum, A.D., W.J. Kraemer, C.J.R. Blimkie, I. Jeffreys, L.J. Micheli, M. Nitka, T.W. Rowland. "Youth Resistance Training: Updated Position Statement from the National Strength and Conditioning Association." *Journal of Strength and Conditioning Research* 23 (August 2009): S60–S79.

Falk, B. and A. Eliakim. "Resistance Training, Skeletal Muscle and Growth." *Pediatric Endocrinology Review* 1 (2003): 120-27.

Falk, B. and G. Tenenbaum. "The Effectiveness of Resistance Training in Children: A Meta-analysis." *Sports Medicine* 22 (1996): 176–86.

Farrey, Tom. "The Power to Motivate Positively." ESPN, March 22, 2003.

Fees, M., et al. "Upper Extremity Weight-Training Modifications for the Injured Athlete." *American Journal of Sports Medicine* 26 (1998): 73–42.

Fleck, S. and W. Kraemer. *Designing Resistance Training Programs.* Champaign, IL: Human Kinetics, 1997.

Flesig, G.S., A. Weber, N. Hassell, J.R. Andrews. "Prevention of Elbow Injuries in Youth Baseball Pitchers." *Current Sports Medicine Report* 8 (2009): 250–54.

FOX Sports. "Report: Violence erupts at hoops tourney," May 31, 2011.

Frank, J. "Lower Extremity Injuries in the Skeletally Immature Athlete." *Journal of the AAOS* 15 (June 2007): 356–66.

Frey, Carol, Keith Feder, and Jill Sleight. "Injury Tracking for West Coast Sports Medicine Foundation, 1998–2008." 2010. Unpublished data.

Garrick, J.G. and R.K. Requa. "Role of External Support in the Prevention of Ankle Sprains." *Medicine & Science in Sports & Exercise* 5 (1973): 200–3.

Gessel, M.L., S.K. Fields, C.L. Collins, R.W. Dick, and R.D. Comstrock. "Concussions among United States High School and Collegiate Athletes." *Journal of Athletic Training* 42 (October–December 2007): 495–503.

Giza, C. and D. Hovda. "The Neurometabolic Cascade of Concussion." *Journal of Athletic Training* 36 (2001): 228–35.

Gross, M.T., A.M. Batten, A.M. Lamm, J.L. Lorren, J.J. Stevens, J.M. Davis, and G.B. Wilkerson. "Comparison of DonJoy Ankle Ligament Protector and Subtalar Sling Ankle Taping in Restricting Foot and Ankle Motion Before and After Exercise." *Journal of Orthopedic & Sports Physical Therapy* 19 (1994): 33–40.

Herlting, D. and R. Kessler. *Management of Common Musculoskeletal Disorders: Physical Therapy Principles and Methods* (third edition). Philadelphia: Lippincott Williams & Wilkins, 1996.

Hickey, J.C., A.L. Morris, L.D. Carlson, and T.E. Seward. "The Relation of Mouth Protectors to Cranial Pressure and Deformation." *Journal of the American Dental Association* 74 (1967): 735–40.

Hobson, Katherine. "Treat Cheerleaders as Athletes, Pediatric Academy Advises." *The Wall Street Journal,* Oct. 22, 2012.

Israel, Michael and Michael O'Brien. Paper presented at the American Academy of Pediatrics annual meeting, New Orleans, October 22, 2012.

Kolata, Gina. "Perks of Cross-Training May End Before Finish Line." *The New York Times,* August 15, 2011.

Lawson, B.R., R.D. Comstock, and G.A. Smith. "Baseball-Related Injuries to Children Treated in Hospital Emergency Departments in the United States, 1994–2006." *Pediatrics* 123 (June 2009): 1028–34.

Light Shields, David, Brenda Light Bredemeier, Nicole M. LaVoi, and F. Clark Power. "The Sport Behavior of Youth, Parents, and Coaches: The Good, the Bad, and the Ugly." *Journal of Research in Character Education* 3 (2005): 43–59.

Maffulli, N. et al. "Aetiology and Prevention of Injuries in Elite Young Athletes." *Medicine & Science in Sports & Exercise* 56 (2011): 187–200.

Maffulli, N., U.G. Longo, and N. Gougoulias. "Sport Injuries: A Review of Outcomes." *British Medical Bulletin* 97 (2011): 47–80.

Mair, Scott, "Arms and the Boy." *The New York Times*, October 21, 2007.

Malina, R. "Weight Training in Youth—Growth, Maturation and Safety: An Evidence-Based Review." *Clinical Journal of Sport Medicine* 16 (2006): 478–87.

Marar, M. et al. "Epidemiology of Concussions among United States High School Athletes in 20 Sports." *American Journal of Sports Medicine* 40 (April 2012): 747–55.

Marshall, W.A. and J.M. Tanner. "Variations in the Pattern of Pubertal Changes in Boys." *Archives of Disease in Childhood* 45 (February 1970): 13–23.

Marshall, W.A. and J.M. Tanner. "Variations in the Pattern of Pubertal Changes in Girls." *Archives of Disease in Childhood* 44 (June 1969): 291–303.

McCrory, P. et al. "Consensus Statement on Concussion in Sport: The 3rd International Conference on Concussion in Sport Held in Zurich, November 2008." *British Journal of Sports Medicine* 43 (2009):i76–i84.

McLain, L.G. and S. Reynolds. "Sports Injuries in a High School." *Pediatrics* 61 (1989): 465–69.

Miller, R.A. et al. "Low-Back Pain in Children: Natural History and Value of Diagnostic Radiologic Studies." *AAP* (2011): abstract 14782.

Mims, Christopher. "Strange but True: Testosterone Alone Does Not Cause Violence." *Scientific American,* July 5, 2007.

Moore, Stephen. "Why Notre Dame Is Back on Top." *The Wall Street Journal,* January 4, 2013.

National Athletic Trainers' Association (NATA). "Collegiate Athletic Injuries—Trends and Prevention." *Journal of Athletic Training* (Spring 2007).

National Collegiate Athletic Association. "Sports Injuries." Accessed June 1, 2013. http://www.ncaa.org.

National Strength and Conditioning Association. "Position Paper on Prepubescent Strength Training." *National Strength and Conditioning Association* J7 (1985):27–31.

Nationwide Children's Hospital, Center for Injury Research and Policy. "High School RIO." Accessed June 1, 2013. http://www.nationwidechildrens.org/cirp-high-school-rio.

Pate, R. R., S. G. Trost, S. Levin, and M. Dowda. "Sports Participation and Health-Related Behaviors among U.S. Youth." *Archives of Pediatric and Adolescent Medicine* 154 (September 2000): 904–11.

Payne, V., J. Morrow, L. Johnson, and S. Dalton. "Resistance Training in Children and Youth: A Meta-Analysis." *Research Quarterly for Exercise and Sport* 60 (1997): 80–88.

Pedowitz, D.I., R. Sudneer, S.G. Parekh, G. Huffman, and B.J. Sennett. "Prophylactic Bracing Decreases Ankle Injuries in Collegiate Female Volleyball Players." *American Journal of Sports Medicine* 36 (2008): 324–27.

Pellman, E.J., M.R. Lovell, D.C. Viano, and I.R. Casson. "Concussion in Professional Football: Recovery of NFL and High School Athletes Assessed by Computerized Neuropsychological Testing–Part 12." *Neurosurgery* 58 (2006): 263–74.

Positive Coaching Alliance. Accessed June 1, 2013. http://www.positivecoach.org.

Powell, J.S., and K.D. Barber Foss. "Injury Patterns in Selected High School Sports: A Review of the 1995–1997 Seasons." *Journal of Athletic Training* 34 (1999): 277–84.

President's Council on Physical Fitness and Sports. "60 Minutes or More a Day, Where Kids Live, Learn, and Play." Accessed June 1, 2013. http://www.fitness.gov.

Purcell, L.K. and C.M.A. LeBlanc. "Pediatric Boxing Participation by Children and Adolescents." Joint Statement, Canadian Paediatric Society and the American Academy of Pediatrics, August 31, 2011. Accessed June 1, 2013. http://www.cps.ca/documents/position/boxing.

Rauh, M.J., A.J. Margherita, S.G. Rice, T.D. Koepsell, and F.P. Rivara. "High School Cross Country Running Injuries: A Longitudinal Study." *Clinical Journal of Sports Medicine* 10 (April 2000): 110.

Safe Kids USA. "Coaching Our Kids to Fewer Injuries: A Report on Youth Sports Safety (April 2012)." Accessed June 1, 2013. http://www.safekids.org.

Safe Kids USA. Accessed June 1, 2013. http://www.safekids.org.

Sampson, N.R. et al. "Knee Injuries in Children and Adolescents: Has There Been an Increase in ACL and Meniscus Tears in Recent Years?" *AAP* (2001): abstract 14815.

Sewall, L. and L.J. Micheli. "Strength Training for Children." *Journal of Pediatric Orthopedics* 6 (1986): 143–46.

Sitler, M.R. and M. Horodyski. "Effectiveness of Prophylactic Ankle Stabilizers on Prevention of Ankle Injuries." *Sports Medicine* 20 (1995): 53–57.

Skinner, B.F. "A Case History in Scientific Method." *American Psychologist* 11 (1956): 221–33.

"Sports-Related Knee Injuries in Children Have Increased Dramatically over the Past Decade." *Science Daily*, October 17, 2011.

Sungot-Borgen, J. and M.K. Torstveit. "Prevalence of ED in Elite Athletes Is Higher Than in the General Population." *Clinical Journal of Sport Medicine* 14 (2004): 25–32.

Tanaka, H., D.L. Costill, R. Thomas, W.J. Fink, and J.J. Widrick. "Dry-land Resistance Training for Competitive Swimming." Medicine and Science in Sports and Exercise 25 (1993): 952–59.

The Renfrew Center Foundation for Eating Disorders. "Eating Disorders 101 Guide: A Summary of Issues, Statistics and Resources." September 2002, revised October 2003.

Thompson, Meghan, Thiphalak Chounthirath, Huiyun Xiang, and Gary A. Smith. "Pediatric Inflatable Bouncer-Related Injuries in the United States, 1990–2010," *Pediatrics* (online, Nov. 26, 2012).

Thurman, D.J., C.M. Branche, and J.E. Sniezek. "The Epidemiology of Sports-Related Traumatic Brain Injuries in the United States: Recent Developments." *Journal of Head Trauma and Rehabilitation* 13 (April 1998): 1–8.

Tropp, H., C. Askling, and J. Gillquist. "Prevention of Ankle Sprains." *American Journal of Sports Medicine* 13 (1985): 259–62.

Verrone Hals, T.M., M.R. Sitler, and C.G. Mattacola. "Effect of a Semi-Rigid Ankle Stabilizer on Performance in Persons with Functional Ankle Instability." *Journal of Orthopedic & Sports Physical Therapy* 30 (2000): 552–56.

Viano, D.C., I.R. Casson, and E.J. Pellman. "Concussion in Professional Football: Biomechanics of the Struck Player–Part 14." *Neurosurgery* 61 (2007): 313–27.

Weisenberger, Lisa. "Limiting the Pitch Count for Young Athletes." American Academy of Orthopaedic Surgeons, April 2011. Accessed June 1, 2013. http://www.aaos.org/news/aaosnow/apr11/clinical6.asp.

Wells, L. and K. Sehgal. "Osgood–Schlatter Disease." In *Nelson Textbook of Pediatrics* (nineteenth edition), edited by R.M. Kliegman, R.E. Behrman, H.B. Jenson, and B.F. Stanton. Philadelphia: Saunders Elsevier, 2011.

White House. "Let's Move." Accessed June 1, 2013. http://www.letsmove.gov.

Wilk, K.E., C. Arriso, J.R. Andrews et al. "Rehabilitation after Anterior Cruciate Ligament Reconstruction in the Female Athlete." *Journal of Athletic Training* 34 (1999): 177–93.

Yeung, M.S., K.M. Chan, C.H. So. "An Epidemiological Survey on Ankle Sprain." *British Journal of Sports Medicine* 28 (1994): 112–16.

Youth Sports Safety Alliance. "Youth Sports Safety Statistics." Accessed June 1, 2013. http://www.youthsportssafetyalliance.org/docs/Statistics-2013.pdf.

Zemper, E. D. and R. W. Dick. "Epidemiology of Athletic Injuries." In *Primary Care Sports Medicine* (second edition), edited by D. McKeag and J. Moeller. Philadelphia, PA: Williams & Wilkins, 2007.

Zucker, N.L., L.G. Womble, D.A. Williamson et al. "Protective Factors for Eating Disorders in Female College Athletes." *Eating Disorders* 7 (1999): 207–18.

Resources

I recommend the following organizations and websites for readers seeking additional information. Please understand that website addresses were current as of the publication date of this book and may change.

General Health and Safety Topics

Start your Internet searches at main portals such as these:
U.S. Department of Health and Human Services
Healthfinder
www.healthfinder.gov

National Library of Medicine
MedlinePlus
www.nlm.nih.gov/medlineplus/

Youth Sports Injuries

American Academy of Pediatrics
Sports Injury Prevention
www.healthychildren.org

CDC
Heads Up: Concussion in Youth Sports
www.cdc.gov/concussion/HeadsUp/youth.html

CDC
Sports Injuries: The Reality
http://www.cdc.gov/safechild/Sports_Injuries/

CDC
ABCs of Raising Safe and Healthy Kids
www.cdc.gov/family/parentabc/index.htm

Education Week
(a helpful website that keeps up-to-date with state concussion laws for student athletes)
www.edweek.org

Safe Kids Worldwide
Safe Kids USA
www.safekids.org

National Institute of Arthritis and Musculoskeletal and Skin Diseases
Childhood Sports Injuries and Their Prevention: A Guide for Parents with Ideas for Kids
www.niams.nih.gov/Health_Info/Sports_Injuries/child_sports_injuries.asp

American Academy of Orthopaedic Surgeons
http://orthoinfo.aaos.org/

Nutrition and Eating Disorders

National Association of Anorexia Nervosa and Associated Disorders
www.anad.org

National Eating Disorders Association
www.nationaleatingdisorders.org

Anorexia Nervosa and Related Eating Disorders (ANRED)
www.anred.com

National Institute of Mental Health (NIMH)
Eating Disorders
www.nimh.nih.gov/health/topics/eating-disorders/index.shtml

National Library of Medicine
MedlinePlus
Eating Disorders
www.nlm.nih.gov/medlineplus/eatingdisorders.html

Female Athlete Triad

Female Athlete Triad Coalition
www.femaleathletetriad.org/

Teens Health from Nemours
http://kidshealth.org/teen/food_fitness/sports/triad.html

Growth

Online calculators can aid in predicting how tall your child will be. These are only estimates:
About.com, Pediatrics
http://pediatrics.about.com/cs/usefultools/l/bl_htcalc.htm

Keep Kids Healthy
www.keepkidshealthy.com/welcome/yahtpredictor.html

About the Authors

Carol Frey, MD, is a board-certified orthopedic surgeon and a diplomate of the American Board of Orthopaedic Surgery. Currently, Dr. Frey is a clinical assistant professor of orthopedic surgery at UCLA and the former chief of the Orthopaedic Foot & Ankle Service at the University of Southern California. She has been a member of the American Orthopaedic Foot and Ankle Society (AOFAS), the American Academy of Orthopaedic Surgeons (AAOS), the Arthroscopy Association of North America (AANA), and California Orthopaedic Association (COA) for over twenty years.

She is a graduate of Stanford University, where she was on the Stanford women's swim team. She is also a graduate of the University of Southern California (USC) School of Medicine. Her training included a residency in orthopedic surgery at the University of California, San Diego (UCSD). In addition, Dr. Frey completed a fellowship in foot and ankle surgery at the Hospital for Joint Disease/NYU in New York City. She also completed a fellowship in orthopedic research at UCSD.

Dr. Frey has served as a board member, program chairman, committee and course chairman, faculty member, task force member, spokesperson, educator, and editor in the field of orthopedic surgery.

She has published more than a hundred manuscripts and book chapters, in addition to editing several medical books on orthopedic, sports medicine, lower extremity, ankle and foot topics, including *Current Practice in Foot and Ankle Surgery*, volumes I and II; *AAOS Essentials of Musculoskeletal Radiology*; and *AAOS Essentials of*

Musculoskeletal Care. Dr. Frey is on the editorial board of *Foot and Ankle International, Biomechanics* and is the foot and ankle section editor for the industry journal *Orthopaedics Today*.

Dr. Frey has been interviewed about her expertise in the field of sports medicine, female athletes, athletic shoes, sports injuries to famous athletes, runner's injuries, and injuries in youth sports by many media outlets, including *ABC News*, the Associated Press, *CBS News*, CNN, *Dateline NBC, Good Morning America*, the *New York Times, People* magazine, *Reader's Digest, Runner's World, USA Today, The Today Show, 20/20*, the *Los Angeles Times, Time, Vogue*, and the *Wall Street Journal*.

This is her first book written for a consumer audience. She and her family live in Manhattan Beach, California. She enjoys open water swimming, watching kids' sporting events, beach volleyball, hiking, and working with high school athletes. She and her husband, Keith Feder, MD, run the West Coast Sports Medicine Foundation, which provides trainers, equipment, education, medical care, and mentoring to over twenty Los Angeles area high school athletic programs. For the past twenty years, the Foundation has provided the same sports medicine care to student athletes in Los Angeles that is delivered to professional athletes.

Jacob Feder is an undergraduate student athlete at the University of California. He played basketball and volleyball for his high school and several elite club travel teams.

Jake is also a serious writer and student who has won awards for his writing from the Hermosa Beach Chamber of Commerce and the Adidas Phenom Basketball Program, where his essay on the person who has inspired him the most was published. That person was his grandfather, Dick Frey, who was a Division 1 basketball player at USC, was awarded the Purple Heart in World War II after being wounded in action in France fighting the Nazis, and won the Helms Medal for Player of the Year in 1940.

Jake has played basketball at the club level since the fourth grade. He was ranked by the AAU for his beach volleyball play and played club volleyball for years. He enjoys working out, staying fit and staying up-to-date on training and diet. He was honored to serve as captain of his varsity basketball squad in high school, received the award for Most Inspirational Player twice, and was selected for the All - League Team. He is looking forward to collegiate basketball and pursing a career in sports medicine and writing.

www.ingramcontent.com/pod-product-compliance
Lightning Source LLC
Chambersburg PA
CBHW060255100426
42742CB00011B/1761